NEW DEVELOPMENTS IN MEDICAL RESEARCH

BOTULINUM TOXINS AND BOTULISM

New Developments in Medical Research

Additional books in this series can be found on Nova's website under the Series tab.

Additional e-books in this series can be found on Nova's website under the e-book tab.

NEW DEVELOPMENTS IN MEDICAL RESEARCH

BOTULINUM TOXINS AND BOTULISM

CHARLOTTE REYNOLDS
EDITOR

New York

Library of Congress Cataloging-in-Publication Data

ISBN: 978-1-63483-384-4

Library of Congress Control Number: 2015945229

Published by Nova Science Publishers, Inc. † New York

Contents

Preface

Botulinism toxins are widely used for the treatment of medical and aesthetic disorders. They are considered the gold standard for the treatment of muscular spasticity and facial dynamics wrinkles. The authors' of this book discuss botulinum toxin resistance in medical and aesthetic arenas; recommendations of dilutions for treatment applications (general recommendations were to inject the toxin diluted, because highly concentrated toxins were believed to be more toxic and dangerous); a novel methodology of transdermal delivery of botulinum toxin with the aid of a dermic pen for hyperhidrosis; emerging treatment options for lower urinary tract symptoms that involve a bladder neck injection of a botulinum toxin; and a discussion on the cases of botulism that arise from consuming certain foods particularly in the Arctic regions.

Chapter 1 – Botulinum toxins are widely used worldwide for the treatment of medical and aesthetic disorders. They are considered the gold standard for the treatment of muscular spasticity and facial dynamic wrinkles. Moreover they are a valid alternative in the treatment of pain and hyperhidrosis. Several adverse events to their applications have been described, being the most frequent hematomas, migraines, palpebral ptosis, ectropion, or lack of response. Resistance to botulinum toxins in the medical field has been described, at higher dosages and short intervals. Nevertheless, resistance to botulinum toxin in aesthetics has been considered traditionally anecdotic. Recent evidence suggests that resistance to botulinum toxins in aesthetics may have higher prevalence than expected. A full analysis of the argument is given with up dated information regarding botulinum toxin resistance in medical and aesthetic arenas; including elements for suspicion and diagnosis, valid alternatives for effective prevention, education and treatment of this misdiagnosed condition.

Chapter 2 – Primary hyperhidrosis is a frequent condition that may deeply impair patient's life quality. Medical and surgical options have been proposed to deal with this disorder. Among the former, botulinum toxins are considered a valid alternative for hyperhidrosis, given its ambulatory minimally invasive procedure. Nevertheless there are several drawbacks to the technique being expensive, temporary, and extremely painful in some areas. Moreover the treatment can give minor or lack of benefits due to insufficient dose or resistance. The anatomical target of the treatment are the sweat glands, nevertheless the majority of the punctures within each treatment reach the deep subcutaneous tissue, with partial loss of the component injected.

A novel methodology of transdermal delivery of botulinum toxin, in non-cross-linked HA emulsion, with the aid of a dermic pen is presented with evident advantages regarding toxin distribution, patient comfort and dosage use in hyperhidrosis.

Chapter 3 – Primary bladder neck dysfunction (PBND) is a condition of lower urinary tract in which the bladder neck does not open enough during voiding; this causes lower urinary tract symptoms (LUTS), which include frequency, urgency, urge incontinence, nocturia (known as "storage symptoms"), hesitancy, incomplete emptying, decrease strength of stream (known as "voiding symptoms"). The true prevalence of this condition is unknown, but many studies showed a marked prevalence between young men with LUTS, accounting for 33-54% of diagnoses; aetiology is still unclear, although there are many theories about this, including muscular and neurological dysfunctions. Diagnosis is made by videourodynamics (VUD), that shows the incomplete or inadequate opening of the bladder neck during voiding, in absence of other causes of anatomical obstruction, such as benign prostatic hyperplasia (BPH). Treatment can be medical or surgical. Medical treatment is based on alpha-blockers, while surgical treatment consists of trans-urethral incision of bladder neck (TUIBN), but these treatments present bothersome adverse effects, such as retrograde ejaculation, especially for young men, and a significant failure rate.

In several recent studies, botulinum neurotoxin-A (BoNT-A) trans-urethral bladder neck injection has been demonstrated to be effective and safe in improving LUTS and uroflow parameters in medically-refractory men with PBND , in absence of significant adverse effects. Although BoNT-A treatment usually needs a re-injection after some months for long-term substained benefits, it's well tolerated, mainly by younger patients who do not tolerate side effects associated with the standard treatments, such as ejaculatory dysfunctions.

Chapter 4 – Traditionally the volume used for botulinum toxin reconstitution has been said to be a matter of personal preference of the physician and not to affect the potency or efficacy of the product. Moreover it was a common belief in Europe that a more concentrated toxin, was more toxic and dangerous. Laboratories general recommendations of dilutions have been considered a guide for treatment applications, but their value has been erratic; changing from product to product and in time within the same product.

The former principles has been tested through differential split face treatments, with different volumes of reconstitution and infiltration. Imaging analysis of the treatments are presented, and discussion of the outcomes is provided. Interestingly identical doses behave different according to volumes variations. New concepts like *minimal responsive dose (MRD), maximum blockage dose (MBD), micro and macro diffusion,* are introduced. Safety issues regarding volume and palpebral ptosis incidence are analyzed.

Chapter 5 – Botulism in the Arctic regions has occurred with some unique food sources. Native fermentation of fish heads, fish eggs, and beaver tail allow proper conditions for botulinum toxin to be elaborated from *Clostridium botulinum.* The consumption of whale meat with the skin attached (*muktuk*) also had been associated with outbreaks of botulism. These unique foods are not consumed anywhere else in the world, and have a disproportionate association with botulism clusters. Cases of botulism from consuming these foods in Alaska and Canada have been described for more than a century. The serotype implicated in botulism from native Arctic foods is almost always type E. Coastal soils from this part of the world are rich in botulism type E. The other distinguishing characteristics of type E botulism is that it can withstand freezing down to 3.5° Celsius, and that it is not saccharolytic, unlike types A and B. Type E botulism has been associated with Norwegian "rakfisk" preparation, a process similar to fermented Arctic foods. Importation of vacuum-packed whitefish from Alaska and Canada has also been associated with sporadic cases of botulism in Europe.

In: Botulinum Toxins and Botulism
Editor: Charlotte Reynolds

ISBN: 978-1-63483-384-4

Chapter 1

Resistance to Botulinum Toxins in Aesthetics

Sebastian Torres Farr, MD
Santa Rita Clinic, Department of Maxilo Facial and aesthetic surgery.
Director of department, Catania, Italy

Abstract

Botulinum toxins are widely used worldwide for the treatment of medical and aesthetic disorders. They are considered the gold standard for the treatment of muscular spasticity and facial dynamic wrinkles. Moreover they are a valid alternative in the treatment of pain and hyperhidrosis. Several adverse events to their applications have been described, being the most frequent hematomas, migraines, palpebral ptosis, ectropion, or lack of response. Resistance to botulinum toxins in the medical field has been described, at higher dosages and short intervals. Nevertheless, resistance to botulinum toxin in aesthetics has been considered traditionally anecdotic. Recent evidence suggests that resistance to botulinum toxins in aesthetics may have higher prevalence than expected. A full analysis of the argument is given with up dated information regarding botulinum toxin resistance in medical and aesthetic arenas; including elements for suspicion and diagnosis, valid alternatives for effective prevention, education and treatment of this misdiagnosed condition.

Introduction

When botulinum toxin (BTX) was first introduced to aesthetics, it was after an observation related to its side effects in the context of blepharospasms treatments. This fact, as with many other drugs permitted the study, development and use of this tool into another area of medicine, such as cosmetic surgery.

The exponential growth of the technique, due to the medical community and patient's interests, increased the knowledge surrounding this molecule, and the safety concerns that called attention at the beginning of the century due to the use of a toxin in aesthetics. Moreover it permitted the study of the adverse events related to the applications. Among the former the most common include; hematomas, migraines, palpebral ptosis, ectropion, or lack of response. A complete list is shown on Table 1.

Any physician with some experience in the aesthetic field understands the importance of patient satisfaction. Whenever we get a patient complaint after a BTX treatment, such as in cases of none or partial response, we face an immediate judge regarding trust, loyalty and professionalism. For these reasons, it is of prime importance to educate or patients concerning the possible causes of their complaint.

Table 1. BTX treatments adverse events

- Pain
- Hematoma, bruising, inflammation
- Headaches
- Palpebral Ptosis
- Pseudo ptosis
- Drug Interaction
- Diplopia
- Asymmetries
- Ectropion
- Allergies
- Unsatisfied Patient
- Muscular Atrophy
- Dysphagia
- Resistance

The causes of lack of response include: drug potency, toxin type, injection technique, unexpressive patients, cold chain alteration, toxin condition, dilution, insufficient dose, unreal expectations and resistance. The causes are summarized in table 2.

With the introduction to the market to new BTX type A, we have found empirically, that even though each toxin claims to have unique and non-interchangeable units, there are toxins that are more powerful than others in clinical response and lasting effect. This has called the attention to the *drug potency* parameter, especially when patients are switched from toxins between different treatments.

Clostridium Botulinum bacteria produces seven serologically distinct types of botulinum neurotoxin (designated as types A, B, C1, D, E, F, and G). All subtypes of toxin act by preventing the release of acetylcholine at the neuromuscular junction. The most potent and used *toxin type* is A. It is clear that when changing the type, very rare condition, we can expect a lesser response to the other types.

Technical errors during the procedure such as intra dermal toxin injections or placement distant to the target muscle, can manifest as lack or partial response in affected areas. Adequate touch ups should guaranteed patient overall satisfaction.

Unexpressive patients are not good candidates for BTX treatments, because they seldom have problems with dynamic wrinkles, and therefore are difficult in perceiving post procedure improvements with the technique.

The *Cold Chain* can be a major concern for BTX that are thermo sensitive. Viability of this type of BTX at room temperature is around 240 hrs. According to Allegan, during BTX production a total of 120 hrs. are consumed at room temperature for production, remaining 120 hrs. for shipping and delivery to destination. Whenever the cold chain is not respected, it is highly probable that part of the vial content is damaged, therefore affecting the performance of it.

To guarantee indemnity storage should be done frozen (-5-8° C) until used and after reconstitution refrigerated at 2-8°C. The use of non-thermo sensitive BTX could be advisable if Cold chain rupture is an issue.

Toxin condition can be altered whenever one of the following is verified: reconstitution >6w (according to Dr. Doris Hexsel publications), alcohol contact with toxin during disinfection, application of ice packs after treatment (favors vasoconstriction and lesser absorption), freezing the toxin after reconstitution (thermic shock damages toxin), or energic shake of the vial after reconstitution. Gentle handling and attention to this details should allow to prevent this event.

Dilution has been traditionally considered as a personal preference of the physician. Nevertheless recent communications by this author have questioned this and open debate regarding the possibility of augmenting the potency of the drug by reducing the amount of solvent in the reconstitution, or better said, by concentrating the toxin. The effects obtained through this are lesser side effects (such as migration) and prompt, more important and long lasting clinical benefits. The author recommends 0,5ml as reconstitution for 125 Speywood Units (Azzalure - Galderma) or 50 Botox units (Vistabex-Allergan) or 1ml for 100 Botox U (Botox-Allergan) or 2 ml for 300 Speywood Units (Dysport-Ipsen).

Doses are gender and individual specific. Most of the textbooks available regarding aesthetic applications of BTX present recipes or treatment forms with practical advices about dose and target muscles. Nevertheless all of this represent general recommendations to orient the clinician to target the specific dose for the specific patient. In this way a correct clinical response is obtained without over or under treatment of the areas involved.

Patient with *unreal expectations* are poor candidates for BTX treatments. A correct clinical history, physical exam and discussion of the procedure with photographs, of previous treatments, will help to rule out them and avoid complications.

Table 2. Possible causes of Lack of Action of BTX

- Drug Potency
- Toxin Type
- Injection technique
- Unexpressive Patients
- Cold Chain
- Toxin condition
- Dilution
- Insufficient Dose
- Un real expectations
- **Resistance**

Resistance to Chemodenervation Definition

This condition is defined as the absence of benefic response and muscular atrophy after BTX treatment, due to an antibody response (of neutralizing antibodies) to the protein content within the product that neutralizes the effect.

The Antibodies Anti-BTX can be:

i. Neutralizing
ii. Non Neutralizing: They do not influence directly on the therapeutic effect, but augment foreign protein charge, increasing potentially the formation of neutralizing antibodies.

All above rank the protein content within a BTX vial as a potential trigger to develop resistance. Although there are areas within the progenitor toxin complex (PTC) that have been identified as more prone to develop neutralizing antibodies, potentially all proteins could develop an immune response that may interfere action and develop resistance. The proteins within a vial are classified in 2 groups:

- Structural proteins: they are present within the toxin complex and include peripheral proteins (hemagglutinin and nonhemagglutinin proteins) and core proteins of the neurotoxin itself. The diagram of the toxin is shown in figure 1.
- The role of these peripheral proteins also known as Nontoxic neurotoxin associated proteins (NAPS) is related to the oral ingestion of the toxin. Non-toxic-non hemagglutinin proteins (NTNHA) protect the progenitor toxin complex against digestive proteases and gastro intestinal acidic ambient, whereas Hemagglutinin proteins (HA) enhance intestinal absorption of it.
- The neurotoxin molecule is a 150kDa protein structure made up of a 100kDa heavy chain and 50kDa light chain held together by a disulfide bond and associated with a zinc atom. The heavy chain has the C-terminus on it and is responsible for the high affinity docking on the presynaptic nerve membrane, being it rapid and irreversible. The light chain is responsible for the intracellular cleavage of proteins required for transmission of acetylcholine across the neuromuscular junction. Regions of the light chain have been recognized by human

anti-toxin antibodies from cervical dystonia patient's immunoresistant to toxin treatment. The antigenic structure of the active toxin recognized by human antibodies relies predominantly on 3 peptides within the light chain named L11, L14 and L18. These 3 antigenic regions reside in close proximity to the belt of the heavy chain. The regions L11 and L18 are accessible in both the free light chain and the holotoxin forms, while L14 appears to be less accessible in the holotoxin. Antibodies against these regions could prevent delivery of the L-chain into the neurons by inhibition of the translocation.

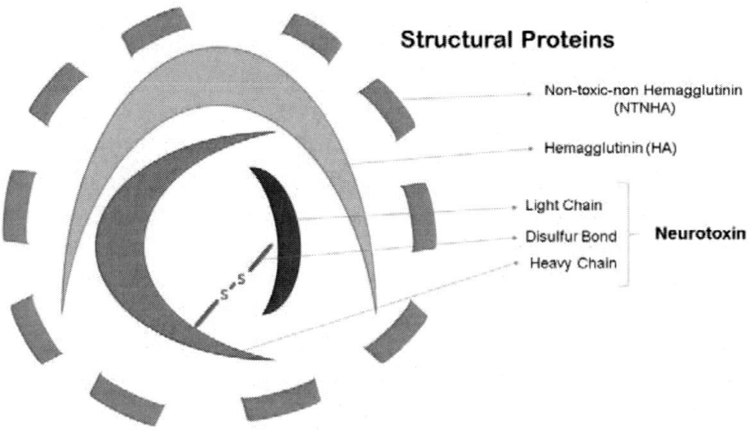

Figure 1. Diagram of Progenitor Toxin Complex evidencing Structural Proteins (NTNHA, HA and neurotoxin).

- Excipients proteins: they are present in most commercial products available in the market in the form of serum albumin, the only exception being the Chinese BTX-A, that uses gelatin as protein stabilizer. This plasmatic transport protein is regularly used in hemodynamic treatments as a volume stabilizer. Moreover it is present in diary and eggs and is susceptible of allergenic response. Nevertheless most of the allergic reactions or intolerances are due to lacto globulin and not serum albumin. The role of this protein in the vials serves especially as protein stabilizer to prevent the adsorption of the toxin to glass and plastic surfaces and probably to maintain the toxin in the target area after being injected. In this case, according to the author theory, would be the principal responsible of limiting micro diffusion. On the other hand, macro diffusion, associated with the most feared complication such as palpebral ptosis, depends on the solvent quantity (or dilution) for the vial preparation.

The other excipients are not important regarding resistance to BTX. Details of the principal characteristics of the most common BTX products available in the market is given in Table 3. Excipients within the vials respect a very strict proportion, and when altered could affect lasting effect.

Table 3. Principal characteristics of most common BTX products available. * CBTX-A, Chinese BoNT/A complex. SA: Serum Albumin, RT: Room Temperature

Product	Toxin type	Lab	Formulation	Units/vial	Excipients	Storage
Azzalure	A	Galderma	Lyophilisate	125 Speywood	125 µg SA 2.5 mg Lactose	2-8°C
Dysport	A	Ipsen	Lyophilisate	300 Speywood	125 µg SA 2.5 mg Lactose	2-8°C
Vistabex	A	Allergan	Vaccum dryed powder	50 Allergan	500 µg SA 0,9 mg NaCl	2-8°C
Botox	A	Allergan	Vaccum dryed powder	100 Allergan	500µg SA 0.9 mg NaCl	2-8°C
Boucuture	A	Merz	Lyophilisate	50 Merz	1000 µg SA Cane Sugar 5 mg	RT
Xeomin	A	Merz	Lyophilisate	100 Merz	1000µg SA 25 mg Sucrose	RT
CBTX-A*	A	Lanzho Institute of Biological Products	Lyophilisate	100	20 mg Gelatin 25 mg Dextran 25 mg Sucrose	-5/-20°C
Myobloc/Neurobloc	B	Solstice	Liquid	5000, 10000, or 20000	500 µg/mL SA 10 nM Na succinate 100 nM Na chloride, Na octanoate pH=5.6	2-8°C

Medical literature has evidenced resistance incidence to be around 0, 3-6%. The first Allergan BTX preparations presented higher protein content within the excipients (Albumin 25ng/vial), which was revised and posteriorly reduced (5ng/vial), dropping resistance concomitantly. The issue was posteriorly forgotten and assumed not to be a problem anymore. As we have just revised protein from all sources within the vial (structural or excipients) may trigger an immune response. Some of the proteins are present in most forms of commercially available preparations (albumin) and some are present in all (the toxin itself). Given this fact and the exponential growth of BTX applications the real actual incidence of the problem is not really clear, and could be higher than expected, especially because you cannot see, what you are not looking for.

BTX Resistance Risk Factors

The principal aspects recognized are:

- Higher doses: this characteristic exposes medical patients to a major risk in comparison to aesthetic applications, and wrongly induced physicians to believe that resistance was not possible in the aesthetic field. As recently demonstrated in the author's publication, resistance in aesthetics is not only possible, but more frequent than expected.
- Short treatment intervals: according to this feature, treatments should only be done every 6 months if possible and touch ups should be limited within the first week and only once.
- Individual predisposition: Some patients are more susceptible than others in resistance development. As with many autoimmune disorders, females seem more prone to be affected, although males usually are treated with higher doses of BTX. A correct clinical history may identify allergic or autoimmune disorders, which could put the patient at increased risk of resistance and could constitute a relative contraindication for the treatment. The exact phenotype of this patients have not been fully understood or identified yet, and genetic tests could give some information about it in the future.

Diagnosis

BTX resistance is based in 2 pillars: clinical suspicion and laboratory tests.

The former is of vital importance as you can only diagnose what you have been trained to see or suspect. Patients present generally upset, after 2 or more BTX treatments in which they refer that the treatment did not gave the expected result, did not work or the intensity or duration of the clinical response was less than expected or experimented in previous treatments.

toxogen Diagnostik GmbH

toxogen GmbH
Feodor-Lynen-Straße 35
30625 Hannover

Order Form

Please test submitted sample(s) for antibodies directed against Botulinum toxin
Type A ☐
Type B ☐ please mark box with a cross where applicable

Patient's particulars

Name:	
First name:	Date of birth:

Treatment

Indication:	
Dose:	Total dose:
Time between injections:	Duration of treatment:

Sender

Doctor:	Phone:
E-Mail:	Fax:
Hospitel:	Ward:
Address:	Postal code:
	Country:

Recipient of invoice (if not identical with sender)

Name:	First name:
Address:	Postal code:
	Country:

Date: ____________________ Signature: ____________________

Feodor-Lynen-Strasse 35
30625 Hannover
Tel 0511 642132-83
Fax 0511 642132-77
labor@toxogen.de
www.toxogen.de

Bankverbindung:
Sparkasse Hannover
BLZ: 250 501 80
Konto: 250 032 78
BIC-/SWIFT: SPKHDE 2H
IBAN: DE77 2505 0180 0025 0032 78

Eingetragen:
Amtsgericht Hannover
HRB-Nr. 56383
USt-ID Nr. DE 189154617

Geschäftsführer:
Prof. Dr. H. Bigalke
Tel.: 0511 642132-83

Figure 2. Resistance Test Form.

The common physician action here is to raise the dose previously used or to change the commercial preparation employed (always staying in BTX-A), increasing both patient anxiety and resistance.

Laboratory test can be clinical, in vivo or in vitro.

Clinical tests are intramuscular measurements of compound potential action and are indirect and not specific.

In vivo tests are considered the gold standard for the diagnosis, since they represent the only FDA approved. The most popular is the bioassay or mouse lethality test. They give quantitative results about the presence of Antibodies in the patient's serum. The test consist in the injection of the suspected patient serum intravenously or intra peritoneal in mouse together with the inoculation of BTX-A. Toxicity or death of the animals is measured and is expected if no or low titers antibodies are present within the patient serum.

It has medium sensitivity and specificity, takes 2-4 days, and is rather expensive (140 Euros). Moreover is complicated (not available in many regions), and has obvious animal rights issues.

The test is available in Hannover Germany in Toxogen Lab (www.toxogen.de). The sample of patient blood (14ml) or serum (5ml) not frozen nor heparinized should be sent in a cold plastic container through express mail. The test form is presented in Figure 2.

In vitro tests include the mouse diaphragm assay (MDA), enzyme-linked immunosorbent assays (Elisa) or the immunoprecipitation assay (IPA).They are not specific and measure only one part of the reaction.

A new in vitro test known as Neuronal Cell-based Botulinum Neurotoxin Assay, based on histological preparations of mouse neural cord is available. It guarantees less animal's death and sufferance (72 tests/animal) and is highly sensitive, specific and safe. For these reasons it may be the test of the future.

A summary of diagnostic tests is given in Table 4.

Prevention

The prophylaxis for resistance development includes: adequate treatment intervals, personalized treatments, minimal effective dose, periodical tests execution, patient education, vast therapeutic arsenal, treatment onset >30y (aesthetic) and to avoid patients with strong allergic or autoimmune phenotype.

Table 4. Diagnostic Test for BTX-A Resistance. SCM: Sternocleidomastoid muscle, ↑: High, ↓: Low, Se: Sensitivity, Sp: Specificity. MDA: mouse diaphragm assay, ELISA: enzyme-linked immunosorbent assays, IPA: immunoprecipitation assay

Type	Name	Characteristics
Clinical	Compound Action Potential	Intramuscular measurements (Frontalis, Extensor Digitorum Brevis, SCM) Indirect ↓ Sp
In Vivo	Mouse Lethality Test	Gold Std, quantitative, FDA approved Medium Se/Sp, complicated Expensive 2-4d Animal rights
In Vitro	MDA Elisa IPA	↓Sp Single phase measurements
	Neuronal Cell-based Botulinum Neurotoxin Assay	Histologic sample of rat neural cord < N° (72 test/animal) & animal suffering ↑ Se/Sp Safer, future

As previously mention, treatment intervals should be 6 months, with the minimum possible interval around 3 months, and touch should be done within the first week after the treatment and only once.

The treatments should be personalized, escaping from traditional formulas, using the minimal effective dose for the target area and avoiding treating areas with little or no mobility or wrinkles (example: procerus muscle in some patients). It is important to keep track on the individual treatment schema and lasting of the clinical effect, as the duration can be the first indicator that there is some resistance development.

In case of suspicion, serologic test should be promptly indicated.

Patients should be informed about this condition and about the other therapeutic alternatives, like bioplasties or laser, which can be combined to avoid the neurotoxin abuse, or "neurotoxin dependent syndrome." In this way we will obtain natural results and maintain facial mobility without wrinkles. The idea is to make patients to consider both; skin quality and facial wrinkles.

Some congress communications in Latin America, have shown the use of BTX in 16y old patients for wrinkles prevention. In this case, although it may be effective, it would expose the patient to a very long way on toxin treatments, and potential resistance. For this reason, in this group wrinkles prevention is advised through a correct cosmetic skin care, sun protection and nutrition. We recommend cosmetic BTX treatments not to be started before the 3rd decade of life.

Finally within the clinical history attention should focus on the autoimmune and allergic phenotypes. Although it is not quite clear, both groups would have an important tendency to develop resistance and should be considered a partial contraindication for BTX applications.

Each case should be discussed and cost benefit decision should be taken with an informed patient.

Treatment

Treatment alternatives include Botulinum toxin type B (BTX-B), medical electronic and infiltrative devices, peelings and cosmetic skin care. A special mention should be given to psychological support for the patient with BTX resistance.

BTX-B, also known as Myobloc (US) or Neurobloc (EC) (Solstice Laboratories) is a toxin of diverse type and although it has a quicker onset than BTX-A is not as potent and the effects will last less. Even though antibody titers tend to diminish in time, new treatments with BTX-A are not suggested. Other important fact to mention is that the drug is intended in Europe for Cervical Dystonia, and not for aesthetic use, so it is very difficult to obtain the product in a private practice setting.

Medical electronic devices embrace non ablative or ablative procedures. Non ablative methodologies include infrared, radiofrequency and localized ultrasounds, only to name a few. Ablative procedures include lasers, like CO2 or erbium.

All above improve collagen synthesis and skin reorganization and may increase dermic thickness reducing visible wrinkles.

Infiltrative devices group bioplasties (to improve skin hydration or metabolism), or needling through derma rollers or dermic pens.

Peelings may enhance skin renewal and tone. They may be superficial, intermediate or deep.

Cosmetic skin care should always be present in our aesthetic practice; it will enhance and maintain our results and is considered to be the single most important measure in skin antiaging. The regimen should consider adequate detergent, day and night time topical preparations and should be adjusted according to the skin type and patients habits.

Finally, it is important to consider the physiological implications of the patient BTX resistant. For many of them, it is considered a major loss, especially if they were used to regular treatments and had experimented its benefits for a long time. It is suggested to listen to the patient fears and to provide alternative options, to avoid helpless or abandon feelings. Psychological support with specialist is advised if during controls, patients is perceived extremely anxious, hesitated or depressed.

Conclusion

Botulinum toxin is one of the best therapeutic weapons available for the treatment of facial dynamic wrinkles and we must, if possible, prevent, suspect, diagnose and treat the presence of resistance, to perpetuate a safe and efficient use of the product for our patients in the future.

References

Atassi MZ, Dolimbek BZ, Jankovic J, et al. Molecular recognition of botulinum neurotoxin B heavy chain by human antibodies from cervical dystonia patients that develop immunoresistance to toxin treatment. *Mol Immunol.* 2008 Sep;45(15):3878-88. doi: 10.1016/j.molimm. 2008.06.031. Epub 2008 Aug 3.

Atassi MZ, Dolimbek BZ, Jankovic J, et al. Regions of botulinum neurotoxin A light chain recognized by human anti-toxin antibodies from cervical dystonia patients immunoresistant to toxin treatment. The antigenic structure of the active toxin recognized by human antibodies. Immunobiology. 2011 Jul;216(7):782-92. doi: 10.1016/j.imbio. 2010.12.009. Epub 2010 Dec 25.

Aun MV, Chung TM, Santos KS, et al. Is age associated with the development of antibodies against botulinum toxin? *Allergol Immunopathol* (Madr).

2013 Jul-Aug;41(4):276-9. doi:10.1016/ j.aller.2012.05.002. Epub 2012 Sep 30.

Bachhuber A, Wagner A, Reichel G, et al. [Proof of botulinum toxin antibodies with the Extensor Digitorum Brevis Test]. *Nervenarzt.* 2008 Aug;79(8):908-11. doi: 10.1007/s00115-008-2470-x.

Brin MF, Comella CL, Jankovic J, et al. Long-term treatment with botulinum toxin type A in cervical dystonia has low immunogenicity by mouse protection assay. *Mov Disord.* 2008 Jul 30;23(10):1353-60. doi: 10.1002/mds.22157.

Chen S. Clinical uses of botulinum neurotoxins: current indications, limitations and future developments. *Toxins* (Basel). 2012 Oct;4(10):913-39. doi: 10.3390/toxins4100913. Epub 2012 Oct 19.

Dowson C, Khan MS, Dasgupta P, et al. Repeat botulinum toxin-A injections for treatment of adult detrusor overactivity. *Nat Rev Urol.* 2010 Dec;7(12):661-7. doi: 10.1038/nrurol.2010.187.

Gil Polo C, Rodríguez Sanz MF, Berrocal Izquierdo N, et al. Blepharospasm and hemifacial spasm: long-term treatment with botulinum toxin. *Neurologia.* 2013 Apr;28(3):131-6. doi: 10.1016/ j.nrl.2012.03.009. Epub 2012 May 29.

Kajbafzadeh AM, Nikfarjam L, Mahboubi AH, et al. Antibody formation following botulinum toxin type A (Dysport) injection in children with intractable bladder hyper-reflexia. *Urology.* 2010 Jul;76(1):233-7. doi: 10.1016/j.urology.2010.03.023. Epub 2010 May 10.

Lowe NJ. Overview of botulinum neurotoxins. *J Cosmet Laser Ther.* 2007;9 Suppl 1:11-6.

Lungu C, Karp BI, Alter K, et al. Long-term follow-up of botulinum toxin therapy for focal hand dystonia: outcome at 10 years or more. *Mov Disord.* 2011 Mar;26(4):750-3. doi: 10.1002/mds.23504. Epub 2011 Feb 1.

Pellett S, Tepp WH, Clancy CM, et al. A neuronal cell-based botulinum neurotoxin assay for highly sensitive and specific detection of neutralizing serum antibodies. *FEBS Lett.* 2007 Oct 16;581(25):4803-8. Epub 2007 Sep 12.

Pérez-Saldaña MT, Tan EK, Burguera JA. Long-term treatment outcome with different formulations of botulinum toxin. *Eur J Neurol.* 2009 Mar;16(3):285-6. doi: 10.1111/j.1468-1331.2008.02508.x.

Pistolesi D, Giannarini G, Stampacchia G, et al. Should we stop using botulinum neurotoxin type a in patients with neurogenic detrusor overactivity after development of secondary resistance? *Eur Urol.* 2011 Oct;60(4):872-3. doi: 10.1016/j.eururo.2011.07.034. Epub 2011 Jul 19.

Ruiz PJ, Castrillo JC, Burguera JA, et al. Evolution of dose and response to botulinum toxin A in cervical dystonia: a multicenter study. *J Neurol.* 2011 Jun;258(6):1055-7. doi: 10.1007/s00415-010-5880-1. Epub 2011 Jan 1.

Torres S, Hamilton M, Sanches E, et al. Neutralizing antibodies to botulinum neurotoxin type A in aesthetic medicine: five case reports. Clin Cosmet Investig *Dermatol.* 2013 Dec 18;7:11-7. doi: 10.2147/CCID.S51938. eCollection 2013.

Yao G, Lee K, GU S, et al. Botulinum neurotoxin A complex recognizes host carbohydrates through its hemagglutinin component. *Toxins* (Basel). 2014 Feb 12;6(2):624-35.doi:10.3390/toxins6020624.

In: Botulinum Toxins and Botulism
Editor: Charlotte Reynolds
ISBN: 978-1-63483-384-4

Chapter 2

Transdermal Delivery of Botulinum Toxins with Dermic Pen for Hyperhidrosis

Sebastian Torres Farr
Santa Rita Clinic Plastic and Maxillo Facial Surgery Department, Catania, Italy

Abstract

Primary hyperhidrosis is a frequent condition that may deeply impair patient's life quality. Medical and surgical options have been proposed to deal with this disorder. Among the former, botulinum toxins are considered a valid alternative for hyperhidrosis, given its ambulatory minimally invasive procedure. Nevertheless there are several drawbacks to the technique being expensive, temporary, and extremely painful in some areas. Moreover the treatment can give minor or lack of benefits due to insufficient dose or resistance.

The anatomical target of the treatment are the sweat glands, nevertheless the majority of the punctures within each treatment reach the deep subcutaneous tissue, with partial loss of the component injected.

A novel methodology of transdermal delivery of botulinum toxin, in non-cross-linked HA emulsion, with the aid of a dermic pen is presented with evident advantages regarding toxin distribution, patient comfort and dosage use in hyperhidrosis

Introduction

Hyperhidrosis is defined as an excessive sweat for the physiologic thermic homeostasis maintenance, which interferes with daily activities and can be a source of great social and psychological distress, that affects 2, 8% of the population.

According to its cause it can be classified in primary (idiopathic) or secondary and depending on its extension is further divided in generalized or focalized (Table 1).

Variable treatments options have been proposed including: topical, oral, medical and surgical options.

Common symptomatology includes: childhood to teenage onset (most frequently), 30-50% of which have familiar background, with no sexual preferences. In this individuals sweating is increased by forty times the average of normal population, reaching levels above 1ml/m^2/min. The most affected regions are axillary, plantar and palmar in combination with other sites. Most affected areas are summarized in table 2.

Diagnosis is mainly based on clinical suspicion, because patients are refractory to ask for advice due to psychological concerns. Common complaints or feelings are daily activities interference, lack of self-confidence, humiliation, shame, sadness, frustration and depression with important social and economic consequences.

Table 1. Hyperhidrosis etiologies

Generalized	Focal
Neurological (Parkinson, spinal cord injury, stroke)	Primary idiopathic
Endocrine (Hypertiroidism, hyperpituitarism, DM, menopause, pregnancy, feocromocitome, carcinoid syndrome, acromegaly)	Frey Syndrome Neuropathy related Spinal cord injury related
Infectious	
CV (shock, heart failure)	
Respiratory Failure	
Drugs	
Toxic (substance abuse, alcohol)	
Oncological (Bone marrow proliferative disorders, Hodgkin disease)	

Table 2. Hyperhidrosis most affected areas and percentages

Affected Area	Percentage
Axillary plus other area	51%
Axillary alone	9,5%
Plantar plus other area	30%
Palmar plus other area	25%
Palmar only	1%
Facial	10%

Physiopathology

Sweat glands (also known as sudoriparous glands) are small tubular structures of the skin that produce sweat. There are two main types that differ in structure, function, secretory product, mechanism of excretion, anatomic distribution, and distribution across species:

- Apocrine sweat glands are mostly limited to the axilla (armpits) and perianal area in humans. They are not significant for thermic homeostasis and their function is related to sexual attraction through pheromones. The secretory portion is larger than eccrine glands (800μm, making them larger overall). They secrete a viscous milky sweat into the pilary canal of the hair follicle.
  They activate and begin functioning during puberty due to hormonal changes, and are most active during stress and sexual excitement.
- Eccrine sweat glands are distributed almost all over the body, in varying densities. Its water-based secretion represents a primary form of cooling in human. They are much smaller than apocrine (secretory coil diameter is 500-700μm), do not extend as deeply into the dermis, and excrete directly onto the surface of the skin.

Diverse stimuli can activate glands. Thermal stimulus activate eccrine glands through acetylcholine, which binds to the gland's muscarinic receptors. Emotional sweating is activated by acetylcholine in eccrine and by adrenaline on both eccrine and apocrine glands. Differences are summarized in table 3.

Table 3. Differences between Apocrine and Eccrine Glands

	Apocrine Gland	Eccrine Gland
Connection to hair follicle	+	-
Secretion	Viscous	Watery
Innervation	Adrenergic (sympathetic) nerves	Cholinergic (parasympathetic) & adrenergic (sympathetic) nerves
Function	Sexual attraction	Thermal regulation
Size and Depth	Bigger and deeper	Smaller and superficial

- Apoecrines sweat glands have characteristics of both previously mention, intermediate in size, found in axilla and perianal region, have ducts opening onto the skin surface. They develop in puberty and can comprise up to 50% of all axillary glands. They secrete the greater amount of watery sweat playing an important role in axillary sweating. Are sensitive to cholinergic activity though they can also be activated via adrenergic stimulation.

The disorder is caused by glands hyper activity (eccrine, apocrines or apoecrines) mainly due to sympathetic hyper tone. As previously mention the principal periglandular nerve neurotransmitter is Acetylcholine, hence the potential benefit of botulinum toxin treatments.

Diagnosis

Clinical suspicion is vital for prompt diagnosis. Lab test aid to rule out secondary causes.

Typically primary hyperhidrosis has onset before 25 years, is diurnal, bilateral, and symmetric. Episodes interfere normal daily activities and recur more than once every week. Positive familiar history is present in more than half of the patients.

Alert Symptoms that should raise suspicion on secondary causes are: fever, nocturnal sweating, weight loss, lymphadenopathies, headaches or palpitations.

Quantitative tests available include: gravimetry, iodine-starch stain and nihidrine.

- Gravimetry: an absorbent paper is weight after a given time. Diagnostic levels for axillary hyperhidrosis are >100mg/5m in men and >50mg/5m in women. Palmar hyperhidrosis is stablished >30mg/m.
- Iodine – starch stain Test: Identifies objectivity the specific sweating area to orient treatment and follow up.

Treatments

Treatment are classified in local or systemic and medical or surgical.

Topical treatments are medical local alternatives, characterized by short acting effect and limited efficacy. For this reason they are limited to minor to mild cases. Among this group aluminum salts are the most effective compound. It generates glandular obstruction, reducing the sweat, but it may cause skin irritation. Systemic treatments include drugs such as: anti cholinergic agents, benzodiazepines, diltiazem, clonidine and Non-steroidal anti-inflammatory drugs.

Anticholinergic agents such as glicopirrolate are effective for mild cases but carry a lot of adverse events including: dry mouth, blur vision, constipation, urinary retention and palpitations.

They can be taken orally or can be transdermally delivered with the aid of Iontophoresis. This ionizing technique allows substance introduction through electricity, being very effective especially for palmar and plantar regions. Should be considered as second option to topical.

Surgical Options include excision, curettage, liposuction, symphatectomy and novel options like needling radiofrequency. The majority is associated with greater morbidity and complications being recommended as the last resort.

Hyperhidrosis and Botulinum Toxin

Toxin inoculation is typically carried out through multiple intradermic injections, being safe and relatively well tolerated. The drug induces a reversible block on cholinergic transmission. Their use is related with greater local and systemic adverse events when compared to aesthetic applications.

A summarize of benefits and drawbacks is given in Table 4.

Axillary Hyperhidrosis and Botulinum Toxin

The treatment is well tolerated with minimal pain with the use of topical anesthesia. Lasting effect varies from 6-7m. Higher dilutions have been traditionally recommended (2,5-5ml per 100U Allergan) to guarantee a better macro diffusion, even though the potency may be affected. Doses vary from 50-200 U Allergan/axilla. Nevertheless, recent concern regarding possible resistance development has given the advice to lower the doses (25U/axilla).

Iodine –starch stain can guide punctures. Generally a grid pattern is design with $1cm^2$ squares. 1-2U (Allergan) are deliver per square with single puncture. The former implies the need of frequent needle change, to maintain needle sharpness. Adverse events related are: inflammation, pain or resistance.

Palmar Hyperhidrosis and Botulinum Toxin

The treatment is extremely painful and traditionally regional blocks are required. The lasting effect typically is around 4-6m. Conventional doses use are between 100-200U (Allergan) per hand. Recent concern regarding possible resistance development has given the advice to lower the doses. The technique is similar to the axillary previously mentioned.

Adverse events include: pain and temporal hand weakness.

Table 4. Benefits and drawbacks of botulinum toxin treatments in Hyperhidrosis

Benefits	Drawbacks
Medical	Temporal (4-8m)
Fast	Expensive
Ambulatory	Compensatory sweating possibility
Decrease sweat up to 80%	Long term effects unknown
	Resistance Potential

Plantar Hyperhidrosis and Botulinum Toxin

Similar pain, dose and duration to palmar. Traditionally need regional blocks prior to the treatment. Success rate smaller than formers.

Facial Hyperhidrosis and Botulinum Toxin

The area mostly affected is the forehead. Additional aesthetic benefits can be observed after treatment.

The Problem

Generally sweat glands consist of a secretory unit consisting of a base rolled into a glomerulum, and a duct that carries the sweat away. The secretory coil or base, is set deep in the lower dermis and hypodermis, and the entire gland is surrounded by adipose tissue.

Skin thickness varies considerably between different races and age-groups, between genders, and different regions of the body. Skin thickness in hyperhidrosis most affected areas varies from 866 μm (forehead) to 1569 μm (sole). Details are given in Table 5.

Average needle size when performing botulinum toxin treatments range from 6 to12,7mm (or even longer) leaving most of the injected toxin deeper to the target of action, the nerves around the glands.

Table 5. Skin thickness in hyperhidrosis most affected areas. E: Epidermis; D: Dermis

	Epidermis (μm)	Dermis (μm)	E + D (μm)
Forehead	94	788	866
Axilla	71	940	1011
Palm	601	746	1349
Sole	637	932	1569

Source: Lee Y, Hwang K. Skin thickness of Korean adults. Surg Radiol Anat (2002) 24: 183–189.

Moreover certain areas that are particularly innervated are very painful and they can express a higher gland density, needing greater amount of punctures. The palm for example has around 370 sweat glands per cm2. In the finger pads, sweat glands are somewhat irregularly spaced on the epidermal ridges. There are no pores between the ridges, though sweat tends to spill into them. The thick epidermis of palms and soles causes the sweat glands to become spirally coiled.

The Device

The dermic pen is a novel medical device characterized by an electronic engine that vibrates and generates a bidirectional movement transferred to a disposable multi needle tip (Derma Needling System, Dermica Laboratories AG, Seoul, Korea) (Figure 1).Vibration can be modulated in depth (from 0, 5 to 2,5) and intensity (1 to 7) to since the benefits of micro needling, altering cutaneous barrier and allowing botulinum toxin or other substances to penetrate the skin. The action of the device over the skin is perceived as a gentle massage, especially if superficial. Moreover it can be used to enhance topical anesthetic absorption prior to treatments. Both actions are particularly useful for the treatment of palmo plantar hyperhidrosis, usually associated with important pain and discomfort by the patients, but can be applied to any other region.

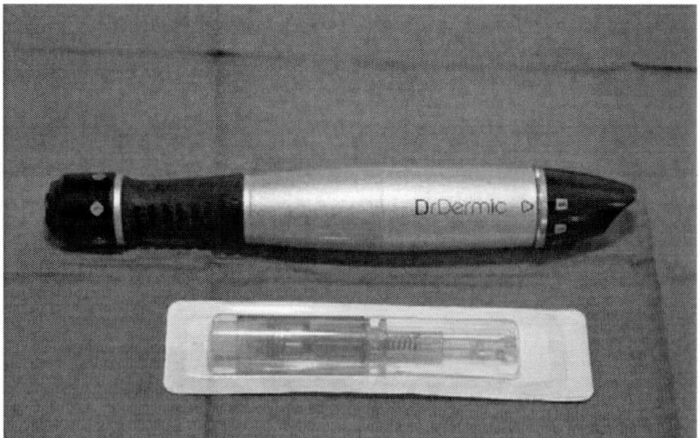

Figure 1. Dermic Pen and disposable needling system.

The Reconstitution

Botulinum toxin is normally prepared with very aqueous sterile solutions (Saline or anesthetics) and if placed over an uneven surface, like the skin, tends to get dispersed and lost rapidly.

As a manner to obtain a more viscous emulsion that will stay longer over the surface of the target area the abobotulinum toxin (125 Speywood Units per vial) is first reconstituted with 0,5ml Saline and posteriorly mixed with 0,5ml non stabilized hyaluronic acid (RRS Hyalift- Aesthetic Dermal SL) (Figure 2) with the aid of two 1ml luerlok syringes and luerlok female to female adaptor (Figure 3). It is vital to obtain a homogeneous emulsion mixing at least 10 times the content of the syringes.

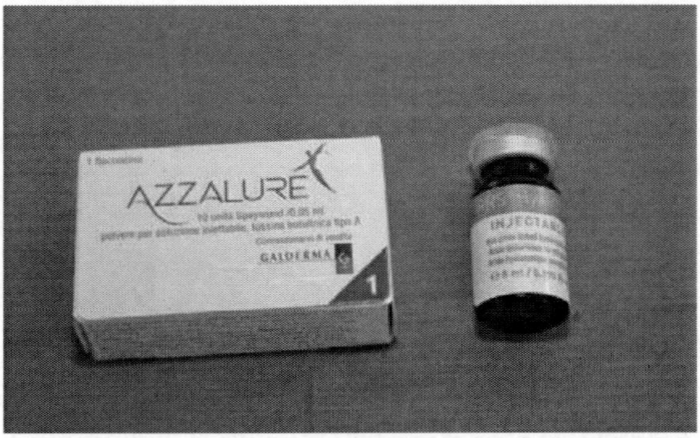

Figure 2. Abobotulinum toxin type A and non-stabilized hyaluronic acid.

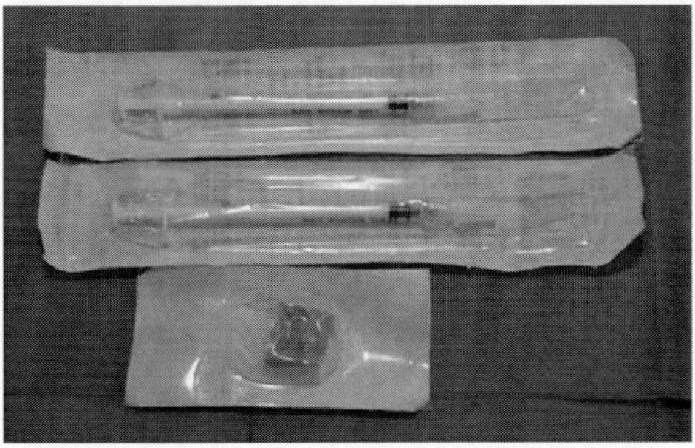

Figure 3. Disposables1ml luerlok syringes and luerlok transfer.

The Treatment

Iodine-starch test should be performed before treatment to orientate the physician about the sweating pattern.

Proper disinfection and cleansing is performed to guarantee removal of dirt and grease. Topical anesthetic ointment is applied generously over the intended surfaces to be treated at least 20 minutes before.

Gently massage is initiated with dermic pen, at 0, 5 depth and speed 7, to enhance anesthetic absorption.

New cleansing and disinfection is carried out to prior to toxin inoculation.

A 0,5ml emulsion (62, 5 Speywood Units) prefilled 1ml luerlok syringe is attached to a small gauge needle to regulate the flow. The dose is enough to treat one area (palm, sole or axilla). In this manner 1 vial is sufficient to treat both hands, feet or armpits. Tiny drops of emulsion are deliver to skin surface and transdermal inoculation is favor with the use of dermic pen (figure 4). Depth is progressively increased from1 to 2 depending on patient tolerance. Emulsion distribution is commanded based on Iodine - starch stain test results (previously performed).

Additional local anesthesia is needed in 10% of palmo-plantar treatments especially around fingers or toes.

Initial results are perceived after 1 week. Occasional retouches are necessary and delivered after 10 days.

Adverse events or reactions described have been greater sensitivity to temperature variations (heat or cold) and prolonged redness (+/-10 days).

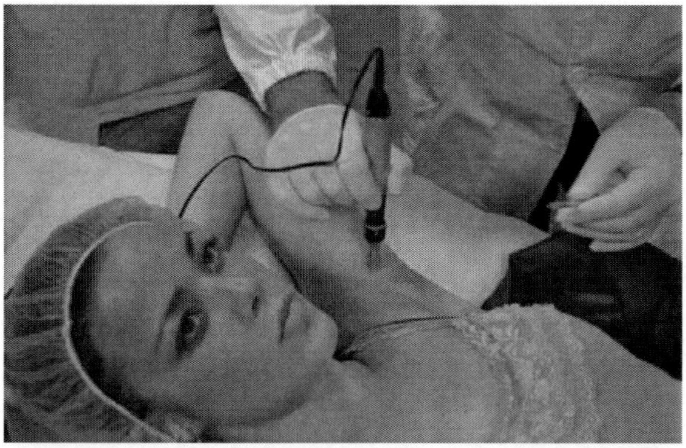

Figure 4. Axillary treatment with dermic pen.

Treatment dose in this manner is reduced to 125 Speywood Units (1 vial) per area affected (both hands, feet or armpits). The drug is delivered at the correct anatomical depth intended and the total dose may be decreased, without altering the result. Effect duration varies between 4-6 months in palms and longer in plantar region. Moreover by decreasing total dose, resistance potential is reduced increasing the lifespan of the treatment.

The treatment is more economical and better tolerated by patients, augmenting compliance and follow up.

References

Benson, RA; Palin, R; Holt, PJ; et al. Diagnosis and management of hyperhidrosis. *BMJ.*, 2013 Nov 25, 347, f6800.

Callejas, MA; Grimalt, R; Cladellas, E. Hyperhydrosis update. *Actas Dermosifiliogr.*, 2010 Mar, 101(2), 110-8.

Chen, S. Clinical uses of botulinum neurotoxins: current indications, limitations and future developments. *Toxins (Basel).*, 2012 Oct, 4(10), 913-39.

Dinulos, JG. Cosmetic procedures in children. *Curr Opin Pediatr.*, 2011 Aug, 23(4), 395-8.

Doft, MA; Hardy, KL; Ascherman, JA. Treatment of hyperhidrosis with botulinum toxin. *Aesthet Surg J.*, 2012 Feb, 32(2), 238-44.

Gordon, JR; Hill, SE. Update on pediatric hyperhidrosis. *Dermatol Ther.*, 2013 Nov-Dec, 26(6), 452-61.

Hosp, C; Naumann, MK; Hamm, H. Botulinum toxin in focal hyperhidrosis. An update. *Hautarzt*, 2012 Jun, 63(6), 469-76.

Iannitti, T; Palmieri, B; Aspiro, A; et al. A preliminary study of painless and effective transdermal botulinum toxin A delivery by jet nebulization for treatment of primary hyperhidrosis. *Drug Des Devel Ther.*, 2014 Jul 14, 8, 931-5.

Ko, EJ; Mun, SK; Oh, IY; et al. Comparison of efficacy and diffusion of three formulations of botulinum toxin type A in two patients with forehead hyperhidrosis. *Clin Exp Dermatol.*, 2014 Jul, 39(5), 673-5.

Kouris, A; Armyra, K; Christodoulou, C; et al. Quality of Life in Patients with Focal Hyperhidrosis before and after Treatment with Botulinum Toxin A. *ISRN Dermatol.*, 2014 Feb 6, 2014, 308650.

Lakraj, AA; Moghimi, N; Jabbari, B. Hyperhidrosis: anatomy, pathophysiology and treatment with emphasis on the role of botulinum toxins. *Toxins (Basel).*, 2013 Apr 23, 5(4), 821-40.

Lee, KY; Levell, NJ. Turning the tide: a history and review of hyperhidrosis treatment. *JRSM Open.*, 2014 Jan 7, 5(1), 2042533313505511.

Lee, Y; Hwang, K. Skin thickness of Korean adults. *Surg Radiol Anat.* (2002), 24, 183–189. DOI 10.1007/s00276-002-0034-5

Naumann, M; Boo, LM; Ackerman, AH; et al. Immunogenicity of botulinum toxins. *J Neural Transm.*, 2013 Feb, 120(2), 275-90.

Naumann, M; Dressler, D; Hallett, M; et al. Evidence-based review and assessment of botulinum neurotoxin for the treatment of secretory disorders. *Toxicon.*, 2013 Jun 1, 67, 141-52.

Shayesteh, A; Nylander, E. Botulinum toxin helps against primary local hyperhidrosis. Good effect—few adverse effects according to a literature review. *Lakartidningen.*, 2011 Nov 23-29, 108(47), 2433-5.

Swartling, C; Brismar, K; Aquilonius, SM; et al. Hyperhidrosis--the "silent" handicap. *Lakartidningen.*, 2011 Nov 23-29, 108(47), 2428-32.

Vergilis-Kalner, IJ. Same-patient prospective comparison of Botox versus Dysport for the treatment of primary axillary hyperhidrosis and review of literature. *J Drugs Dermatol.*, 2011 Sep, 10(9), 1013-5.

Walling, HW; Swick, BL. *Treatment options for hyperhidrosis Am J Clin Dermatol.*, 2011 Oct 1, 12(5), 285-95.

In: Botulinum Toxins and Botulism
Editor: Charlotte Reynolds
ISBN: 978-1-63483-384-4

Chapter 3

Bladder Neck Injection of Botulinum Toxin: An Emerging Treatment Option for Lower Urinary Tract Symptoms due to Primary Bladder Neck Dysfunction

Emilio Sacco*[*]*, MD, PhD and Riccardo Bientinesi, MD
Urology Department, "Agostino Gemelli" Academic Hospital,
Catholic University of Sacred Heart, Rome, Italy

Abstract

Primary bladder neck dysfunction (PBND) is a condition of lower urinary tract in which the bladder neck does not open enough during voiding; this causes lower urinary tract symptoms (LUTS), which include frequency, urgency, urge incontinence, nocturia (known as "storage symptoms"), hesitancy, incomplete emptying, decrease strength of stream (known as "voiding symptoms"). The true prevalence of this condition is

[*] Email: emilio.sacco@gmail.com

unknown, but many studies showed a marked prevalence between young men with LUTS, accounting for 33-54% of diagnoses; aetiology is still unclear, although there are many theories about this, including muscular and neurological dysfunctions. Diagnosis is made by videourodynamics (VUD), that shows the incomplete or inadequate opening of the bladder neck during voiding, in absence of other causes of anatomical obstruction, such as benign prostatic hyperplasia (BPH).

Treatment can be medical or surgical. Medical treatment is based on alpha-blockers, while surgical treatment consists of trans-urethral incision of bladder neck (TUIBN), but these treatments present bothersome adverse effects, such as retrograde ejaculation, especially for young men, and a significant failure rate.

In several recent studies, botulinum neurotoxin-A (BoNT-A) trans-urethral bladder neck injection has been demonstrated to be effective and safe in improving LUTS and uroflow parameters in medically-refractory men with PBND , in absence of significant adverse effects. Although BoNT-A treatment usually needs a re-injection after some months for long-term sustained benefits, it's well tolerated, mainly by younger patients who do not tolerate side effects associated with the standard treatments, such as ejaculatory dysfunctions.

Primary Bladder-Neck Dysfunction

Primary bladder neck dysfunction (PBND), first described in men by Marion in 1933 [1], is a condition in which the bladder neck fails to open enough during voiding, thus resulting in a weak urinary stream, in absence of another anatomical obstruction, such as that caused by benign prostatic hyperplasia (BPH) in men or genitourinary prolapse in women. PBND was also described in women in 1984 by Diokno et al. [2] and in 1987 by Axelrod and Blaivas [3]; both described this condition in 3 women.

Epidemiology and Aetiopathogenesis

The true prevalence of PBND in male and female population is unknown. In a retrospective study, Kaplan and coll. reported a 54% of incidence of PBND in a group of men younger than 50 years affected by chronic voiding dysfunction [4]. Other studies on men younger than 50 years with LUTS reported a prevalence of PBND between 41% and 47% [5, 6]. Data about the prevalence of PBND in women are poor, with just a few cases being described

in literature. The exact etiology of PBND has not yet been clearly elucidated. There are various theories about the etiology of this condition, including the initial Marion's theory, sustaining the presence of structural changes at the bladder neck, such as a fibrous narrowing or hyperplasia [1]. In 1959, Leadbetter suggested as aetiopathogenesis a fault of dissolution of mesenchyme at the bladder neck or inclusion of abnormal amounts of non-muscular connective tissue, resulting in hypertrophic smooth muscle, fibrous contractures, and inflammatory changes at the bladder neck [7]. In 1973, Turner-Warwick and coll. first described an inadequate opening of bladder neck during micturition due to an abnormal morphological disposition of the detrusor-trigonal smooth muscle [8].

Clinical Presentation and Diagnosis

Clinically, PBND may present with a variety of symptoms, which are generally classificated in voiding symptoms and storage symptoms, the so called *lower urinary tract symptoms* (LUTS). Voiding symptoms, also known as obstructive symptoms, include hesitancy, decreased force of stream, intermittent stream, incomplete emptying; storage symptoms, otherwise called irritative symptoms, include nocturia, frequency, urgency, urge incontinence. These symptoms may present alone or in combination [5-7]. In some cases, initial presentation may be an acute urinary retention. Many conditions bring on similar symptoms as bladder neck obstruction; these conditions include urinary tract infections, benign prostatic hyperplasia and neurogenic bladder [9]. PBND is a videourodynamic diagnosis [6, 10, 11]. Videourodynamic studies show characteristically a relative high-pressure, low-flow voiding with radiographic evidence of obstruction at the bladder neck with relaxation of the striated sphincter and no evidence of distal obstruction. In men, the meaning of *high pressure* and *low flow* in PBND has not been universally defined.

In various series on PBND, detrusor pressure at maximum flow ranges from 20 cm H2O to 70 cm H2O with maximum flow rates (Qmax) of less than 15 mL/s [9, 12]. Recently, Nitti et coll. categorized PBND in three types: the classic, with high detrusorial pressure and low flow; the normal pressure-normal flow type, with narrowing at the bladder neck; the delayed opening of the bladder neck type [5]. All three these classifications represent bladder neck dysfunction causing obstruction. In some cases, cystoscopy may be useful in finding other urethral problems, but is not indicated for PBND diagnosis.

Standard Treatment Options

Treatment options for PBND include pharmacological therapy and surgical intervention. The base of the pharmacological therapy for PBND are α-blockers. Although much of their effects are presumed to involve the bladder neck smooth muscle, α-blockers may also affect the bladder via local or central mechanisms, as is assumed to be the case in BPH treatment. However, only variable success has been reported for α-blocker therapy for PBND, contrary to BPH treatment. Most studies in literature are small, nonrandomized, and noncontrolled, with no consistency in type or dosage of drug. In addition, there are no reported placebo-controlled studies, and outcomes have been variable [12-15].

Surgical treatment of PBND consists in unilateral or bilateral transurethral incision of the bladder neck (TUIBN). In 1973, Turner-Warwick et coll. first introduced the concept of transurethral bladder neck incision [8]. Since then, several studies showed that TUIBN is the most effective treatment for PBND [16, 17]. Bladder neck incision and resection may also be used to treat PBNO in women, as showed by Axelrod and Blaivas in their study, where they reported success in all treated cases [3] and by Zhang et al in a most recent study [18]. The main, bothersome, side effect of TUIBN in men is postoperative retrograde ejaculation, which occurs in 27-100% of patients undergoing this procedure [12, 17]. Performing an unilateral incision or preserving a portion of the supramontanal tissue during the procedure may reduce the postoperative incidence of retrograde ejaculation [16, 19], but these data should be confirmed by greater studies.

Botulinum Toxin Injection Therapy

Botulinum toxin A (BoNT-A), the clinically most relevant from seven known BoNT subtypes, is a 150-kDa molecule, consisting of a heavy and a light chain. The known mechanism of action on striated skeletal muscles is the inhibition of acetylcholine (Ach) release at motoric axon terminals; in particular, it prevents exocytosis of the neurotransmitter Ach into the synaptic space [20, 21]. Thus, it causes a flaccid muscle paralysis, which is however of limited duration (months) due to re-sprouting of the axon terminals [21, 22].

Onabotulinum toxin A (onabotA, Botox®), abobotulinum toxin A (abobotA, Dysport®), and incobotulinum toxin A (incobotA) are available BoNT-As for clinical use [23, 24]. BoNT-A has long been used in Neurology for the treatment of focal spasticity of striated skeletal muscles; in 1998 it has been introduced into the field of Urology by Dykstra et coll. for the treatment of detrusor-sphincter dyssynergia [25]. In 2000, the first BoNT-A application in the smooth detrusor muscle in patients with neurogenic detrusor overactivity was described by Schurch et coll. [26], followed in 2003 by the first results on the intraprostatic injection of BoNT/A for the treatment of BPH by Maria et al. [27].

Actually in urology BoNT-A is routinely used in different conditions [28], and has received regulatory approval for use in neurogenic detrusor overactivity (NDO) and overactive bladder (OAB) refractory to conservative and pharmacological treatments, injected into the detrusor muscle transurethrally [29, 30-32]. Its use in the treatment of other LUTS causes, such as BPH [27], bladder pain syndrome (BPS) [28], and detrusor sphincter dyssynergia (DSD) [25] is still *off-label.*

In 2008 Sey Kiat Lim first described in a pilot study the use of BoNT-A in the treatment of PBND [33]. In this prospective, non-blinded and uncontrolled study, authors enrolled 8 young patients (mean age 36,9 years) diagnosed with PBND and previous treated with α-blockers with or without anticholinergics, without success; diagnosis was made by VUD, and all patients had a maximum urinary flow rate (Qmax) <15 ml/sec and moderate/severe LUTS (IPSS>15). All patients were treated with Botox® (Allergan) diluted at 10U/ml with saline and injected transurethrally with a 22 Ch rigid cystoscope in 10 different sites in the bladder neck and in the lateral prostatic lobes (1 ml per injection). Authors defined the success rate as a reduction of IPSS >50% and an increase of the Qmax >3 ml/sec. In the postoperative evaluation, authors observed a significative reduction in IPSS in 7 of 8 patients at 1 week until 4 months after treatment, with a significative increase in Qmax >3 ml/sec in 6 of 8 patients until 16 weeks. These results lost their statistical significance after 16 weeks, while symptoms appeared to recur after 8 months. All patients well tolerated the treatment. Potential side effects like urinary retention, urinary incontinence, gross hematuria, urinary tract infection, or systemic weakness were not reported. In addition, no patient reported any decrease in ejaculatory volume or ejaculatory dysfunction, such as retrograde ejaculation.

In 2009 Jing-Liang Chen et al. treated 30 patients (aged from 35 to 78 years) with BOO due to PBND with transurethral injection of 100U of BoNT-A (Botox®, Allergan) diluted in 10 ml of saline [34]. They performed transurethrally with a rigid cystoscope 10 injections in 10 different sites in the bladder neck and in the prostatic urethra (1 ml per injection). After treatment, authors evaluated IPSS, Qmax, quality of life (QoL) index at 1, 3 and 6 months; moreover, Patients reported a subjective satisfaction score on a global satisfaction scale (ranging from 0 –none- to 3 –excellent). After treatment, IPSS improved significantly at 1 and 3 months, but not at 6 months. Qmax increased at 1 and 3 months and remained improved at 6 months. At 1 month after treatment, the overall satisfaction rate from the treatment was of 86.6% and remained the same at 3 months, but decreased to 60% at 6 months. In this series, immediately after BoNT-A injection, two patients experienced mild pain on micturition, one had gross hematuria and one had acute urinary retention that resolved after catheterization for 2 days. No urinary tract infection or chronic urinary retention developed in any patient.

In 2013 Sacco et al. performed a prospective study treating 30 patients with videourodynamic diagnosis of PBND with intracervical BoNT-A [35]. They injected 200 U of BoNT-A (Botox®, Allergan) diluted in 4ml of saline (50 U/ml), transurethrally at four sites (3-6-9-12 o'clock, 1 ml/site) into the bladder neck, at about 1 cm from bladder-neck edge, using a 23 gauge needle through a 22F rigid cystoscope. Patients were meanly aged 18–50 years, diagnosed with PBND on VUDS, refractory to a-blockers with or without anticholinergics for at least 3 months, as defined by persistent moderate to severe LUTS (IPSS > 15) and Qmax < 15 ml/sec. All patients had a wash-out phase from previous pharmacological therapies of 28 days before treatment. Patients were evaluated at 2, 6, 9 and 12 months after therapy. A reduction in mean total IPSS from baseline was observed at all postoperative evaluations, but it did not achieve statistical significance at 12 months. The rate of change from baseline in total IPSS values appeared to be very large in the early follow-up period, however, it showed a progressive downtrend later on. Likewise, a reduction from baseline in mean values of both storage-IPSS and voiding-IPSS was observed at all postoperative evaluations, but it failed to achieve statistical significance at 12 months. The increase in mean Qmax values from baseline remained statistically significant until 9 months, although a continuous downtrend was observed after the early increase. In this study, authors first provided an insight into the effect of BoNT-A from the patient's perspective, using PROs (patient reported outcomes) questionnaires; the assessment of PROs showed that satisfaction with the efficacy of the treatment on LUTS control was reported by 80%, 70%, and 46.7% of patients at 2, 6, and 9 months, respectively, and 41.4% was still satisfied at 12 months. Likewise, 80.0%, 73.3%, and 60.0% of patients expressed overall satisfaction at 2, 6, and 9 months, respectively, and 44.8% still reported satisfaction at 12 months. In all, 23 (79.3%) patients would repeat the same treatment in the same circumstances and 25 (86.2%) patients would recommend the treatment to another person with the same problem. In this study, during treatment and follow-up, no systemic adverse effects related to the treatment were reported. Postoperatively, 19 (63.3%) and 13 (43.3%) patients reported painful micturition and mild gross hematuria, respectively, but both problems resolved spontaneously in 24 hr. Four (13.3%) patients experienced postoperative complete urinary retention requiring overnight urethral catheterization.

The results of these studies showed that transurethral injection of BoNT-A into the bladder neck is an effective treatment in younger patients with medically refractory PBND. In their study [33], Sey Kiat Lym et coll. first postulated that BoNT-A effects might result in relaxation or even atrophy of the bladder neck, reducing the delay in bladder-neck opening and improving flow result, on the basis of the two main theories of BND, that revolve around an extension of the external sphincter and increased sympathetic tone at the bladder neck [36]. Many studies involving BoNT-A for various voiding dysfunction conditions showed that the mean duration of action of BoNT-A is about 8–11 months [37, 38], which largely concurred with the findings of the mentioned studies. Results of the three studies are overlapping, with some differences, and comparable favorably also with those reported in studies on TUIBN [9, 13]; The TUIBN has the advantage of sustained long-term benefit without the need of re-do procedures. However, the main trouble with this invasive treatment is the development of retrograde ejaculation in 11–27% of patients [9]. Sacco et al. used a double dose of BoNT-A, with the assumption that a higher dose would improve the clinical efficacy; the same dose has been largely used in BPH patients' series without increasing adverse effects [39]. On the other hand, they used a small dilution volume in order to avoid routine catheterization and to limit the risk of postoperative urinary retention [33]. In every case, as showed by results of the studies, the treatment is safe and not associated to ejaculatory dysfunctions. The generalizability of the showed findings is limited by the *openlabel*, non-comparative design of the studies, with lack of a placebo arm. Consequently, the results of these studies, though encouraging, should not be embraced into regular practice as such. However, even if *off-label*, in patients who are refractory to medical treatment for BPH, BoNT-A injection for bladder neck might be an effective option; repeated treatments are required for long-term sustained effectiveness and patients should be informed of the time-limited effectiveness.

References

[1] Marion G: Surgery for the neck of the bladder. *Br. J. Urol.* 1933; 5:351-357.

[2] Diokno AC, Hollander JB, Bennett CJ. Bladder neck obstruction in women: a real entity. *J. Urol.* 1984;132:294-298.

[3] Axelrod SL, Blaivas JG. Bladder neck obstruction in women. *J. Urol.* 1987;137:497-499.

[4] Kaplan SA, Ikeguchi EF, Santarosa RP, et al: Etiology of voiding dysfunction in men less than 50 years of age. *Urology* 1996; 47:836-839.

[5] Nitti VW, Lefkowitz G, Ficazzola M, Dixon CM: Lower urinary tract symptoms in young men: Videourodynamic findings and correlation with noninvasive measures. *J. Urol* 2002; 168:135-138.

[6] Wang CC, Yang SSD, Chen YT, Hsieh JH: Videourodynamics idenifies the causes of young men with lower urinary tract symptoms and low uroflow. *Eur. Urol.* 2003; 43:386-390.

[7] Leadbetter GW, Leadbetter WF. Diagnosis and treatment of congenital bladder neck obstruction in children. *N. Engl. J. Med.* 1959;260:633.

[8] Turner-Warwick R, Whiteside CG, Worth PHL, et al. A urodynamic view of the clinical problems associated with bladder neck dysfunction and its treatment by endoscopic incision and transtrigonal posterior prostatectomy. *Br. J. Urol.* 1973;45:44-59.

[9] Kaplan SA, Te AE, Jacobs BZ. Urodynamic evidence of vesical neck obstruction in men with misdiagnosed chronic nonbacterial prostatitis and the therapeutic role of endoscopic incision of the bladder neck. *J. Urol.* 1994;152:2063-2065.

[10] Nitti VW, Lefkowitz G, Ficazzola M, Dixon CM. Lower urinary tract symptoms in young men: videourodynamic findings and correlation with non-invasive measures. *J. Urol.* 2002;168:135-138.

[11] Chung-Cheng Wang, Stephen Shei Dei Yang. Diagnosis and Treatment of Primary Bladder Neck Obstruction in Young Men. *Incont. Pelvic. Floor Dysfunct* 2007;1:9-11.

[12] Yang SSD, Wang CC, Hseih CH, Chen YT. α1-adrenergic blockers in young men with primary bladder neck obstruction *J. Urol.* 2002;168:571-574.

[13] Trockman BA, Gerspach J, Dmochowski R, Haab F, Zimmern PE, Leach GE: Primary bladder neck obstruction: Urodynamic finding and treatment results in 36 men. *J. Urol.* 1996; 156: 1418-1420.

[14] Mishra VK, Kumar A, Kapoor R, Srivastava A, Bhandari M: Functional bladder neck obstruction in males: A progressive disorder? *Eur. Urol.* 1992; 22:123-129.

[15] Yamanishi T, Yasuda K, Sakakibara R, et al. The effectiveness of terazosin, an α1-blocker, on bladder neck obstruction as assessed by urodynamic hydraulic energy. *BJU Int.* 2000;85:249-253.

[16] Yang SS, Tsai YC, Chen JJ, Peng CH, Hsieh JH, Wang CC. Modified transurethral incision of the bladder neck treating primary bladder neck obstruction in young men: a method to improve voiding function and to preserve antegrade ejaculation. *Urol. Int.* 2008;80(1):26-30.

[17] Huckabay C, Nitti VW. Diagnosis and treatment of primary bladder neck obstruction in men. *Curr. Urol. Rep.* 2005;6(4):271-5.

[18] Zhang P, Wu ZJ, Xu L, Yang Y, Zhang N, Zhang XD. Bladder neck incision for female bladder neck obstruction: long-term outcomes. *Urology*. 2014 Apr;83(4):762-6.

[19] Kochakarn W, Lertsithichai P. Unilateral incision for primary bladder neck obstruction: symptom relief and fertility preservation. *World J. Urol.* 2003;21:159-162.

[20] Lam SM. The basic science of botulinum toxin. *Facial Plast. Surg. Clin. North Am.* 2003; 11:431–438.

[21] Montal M. Botulinum neurotoxin: a marvel of protein design. *Annu. Rev. Biochem.* 2010; 79:591–617.

[22] MacKenzie I, BurnstockG,Dolly JO. The effects of purified botulinum neurotoxin type A on cholinergic, adrenergic and non-adrenergic, atropine-resistant autonomic neuromuscular transmission. *Neuroscience* 1982;7:997–1006.

[23] Chancellor MB, Fowler CJ, Apostolidis A, et al. Drug Insight: biological effects of botulinum toxin A in the lower urinary tract. *Nat. Clin. Pract. Urol.* 2008; 5:319–328.

[24] Mangera A, Andersson KE, Apostolidis A, et al. Contemporary management of lower urinary tract disease with botulinum toxin A: a systematic review of botox (onabotulinumtoxinA) and dysport (abobotulinumtoxinA*). Eur. Urol.* 2011;60:784–795.

[25] Dykstra DD, Sidi AA, Scott AB, et al. Effects of botulinum A toxin on detrusorsphincter dyssynergia in spinal cord injury patients. *J. Urol.* 1988; 139:919–922.

[26] Schurch B, Schmid DM, Stohrer M. Treatment of neurogenic incontinence with botulinum toxin A. *N. Engl. J. Med.* 2000; 342:665.

[27] Maria G, Brisinda G, Civello IM, et al. Relief by botulinum toxin of voiding dysfunction due to benign prostatic hyperplasia: results of a randomized, placebo-controlled study. *Urology* 2003; 62:259–264.
[28] Mangera A, Apostolidis A, Andersson KE, Dasgupta P, Giannantoni A, Roehrborn C, Novara G, Chapple C. An updated systematic review and statistical comparison of standardised mean outcomes for the use of botulinum toxin in the management of lower urinary tract disorders. *Eur. Urol.* 2014;65(5):981-90.
[29] Dmochowski R, Chapple C, Nitti VW, et al. Efficacy and safety of onabotulinumtoxinA for idiopathic overactive bladder: a double-blind, placebo controlled, randomized, dose ranging trial. *J. Urol* 2010; 184:2416–2422.
[30] Cruz F, Herschorn S, Aliotta P, Brin M, Thompson C, LamW, et al. Efficacy and safety of onabotulinumtoxinA in patients with urinary incontinence due to neurogenic detrusor overactivity: a randomised, double-blind, placebo-controlled trial. *Eur. Urol.* 2011;60(4):742–50.
[31] Ginsberg D, Gousse A, Keppenne V, Sievert KD, Thompson C, Lam W, et al. Phase III efficacy and tolerability study of onabotulinumtoxinA for urinary incontinence from neurogenic detrusor overactivity. *J. Urol.* 2012;187(6):2131–9.
[32] Rovner E, Dmochowski R, Chapple C, Thompson C, Lam W, Haag-Molkenteller C. OnabotulinumtoxinA improves urodynamic outcomes in patients with neurogenic detrusor overactivity. *Neurourol. Urodyn.* 2013.
[33] Sey Kiat Lim, Pearllyn L.C. Quek. Intraprostatic and Bladder-Neck Injection of Botulinum A Toxin in treatment of males with bladder-neck dyssynergia: A Pilot Study. *Eur. Urol.*, 2008; 53, 620–627.
[34] Jing-Liang Chen, Chia-Yen Chen, Hann-Chorng Kuo. Botulinum Toxin A Injection to the Bladder Neck and Urethra for Medically Refractory Lower Urinary Tract Symptoms in Men Without Prostatic Obstruction. *J. Formos Med. Assoc.* 2009 Dec;108(12):950-6.
[35] Sacco E, Tienforti D, Bientinesi R, D'Addessi A, Racioppi M, Pinto F, Totaro A, Vittori M, D'Agostino D, Bassi P. OnabotulinumtoxinA injection therapy in men with LUTS due to primary bladder-neck dysfunction: objective andpatient-reported outcomes. *Neurourol. Urodyn.* 2014;33(1):142-6.
[36] Elbadawi A. Ultrastructure of vesicourethral innervation. Postganglionic axoaxonal synapses in intrinsic innervation of the vesicourethral

lissosphincter: a new structural and functional concept in micturition. *J. Urol.* 1984;131:781–90.

[37] Schmid D, Sauermann P, Werner M, et al. Experience with 100 cases treated with botulinum–a toxin injections in the detrusor muscle for idiopathic overactive bladder syndrome refractory to anticholinergics. *J. Urol.* 2006;176:177–85.

[38] Apostolidis A, Dasgupta P, Fowler CJ, et al. Proposed mechanism for the efficacy of injected botulinum toxin in the treatment of human detrusor overactivity. *Eur. Urol.* 2006;49:644–50.

[39] Oeconomou A, Madersbacher H. Botulinum neurotoxin A for benign prostatic hyperplasia. *Curr. Opin. Urol.* 2010;20:28.

In: Botulinum Toxins and Botulism
Editor: Charlotte Reynolds
ISBN: 978-1-63483-384-4

Chapter 4

Botulinum Toxins: A Matter of Dilution

Sebastian Torres Farr
Santa Rita Clinic Plastic and Maxillo Facial Surgery Department
City/Country: Catania, Italy

Abstract

Traditionally the volume used for botulinum toxin reconstitution has been said to be a matter of personal preference of the physician and not to affect the potency or efficacy of the product. Moreover it was a common belief in Europe that a more concentrated toxin, was more toxic and dangerous.

Laboratories general recommendations of dilutions have been considered a guide for treatment applications, but their value has been erratic; changing from product to product and in time within the same product.

The former principles has been tested through differential split face treatments, with different volumes of reconstitution and infiltration. Imaging analysis of the treatments are presented, and discussion of the outcomes is provided. Interestingly identical doses behave different according to volumes variations. New concepts like *minimal responsive dose (MRD), maximum blockage dose (MBD), micro and macro diffusion,* are introduced. Safety issues regarding volume and palpebral ptosis incidence are analyzed.

Introduction

Toxin reconstitution has been traditionally considered a minor factor, irrelevant regarding drug potency or action. The former has encouraged the producing companies to give erratic recommendations about the volume to be used with each particular product, changing in between different brands and within each product in time. A common belief has been that reconstitution volume depends mainly on physicians' personal manual preferences, or thumb sensitivity or dexterity. Moreover it has been proposed that toxin diffusion is principally related to the synthesis process.

Following its appearance in Europe the term toxin was associated with possible harmful events regarding the dose and concentration administered. General recommendations were to inject the toxin diluted, because highly concentrated toxins were believed to be more toxic and dangerous.

To test all above a clinical study was conducted that applied differential split face treatments, with different reconstitutions for each vial, and different volumes injected per side.

Clinical Study

Five female patients age interval 40-50 years, with non-prior exposure to botulinum toxin were given differential treatments for right and left hemi face, regarding the reconstitution volume of the vial and the total volume injected per side. An identical amount of toxin Units was given per treatment area on each side.

Side assignation was random. The study was independent with no financial support from any company. The product used was AboBotulinum toxin A (Azzalure® – Galderma) 125 Speywood Units per vial (Ipsen Pharmaceuticals). All treatments were performed for free by the same practitioner. A special informed consent was given to specify possible differential responses and asymmetries. The muscles treated included orbicularis oculi, corrugators and frontal. Muscles of the midline were not treated. A photographic assessment was performed before and after the treatments. Facial analysis was executed at rest and in motion. Retouches were given as necessary to achieve symmetry. Each patient was its own case and control. Dilutions volume ranged from 0, 25 to 1,5ml for the 125 Speywood Units vial.

Patient 1, paralleled 0,5 vs 1 ml on dilution; patient 2, compared 1 vs 0,25 ml; patient 3, 0,25 vs 1,5ml; patient 4, tested 1,5 vs 0,25 ml and patient 5, 0,25 vs 0,5ml. The total amount of Speywood Units per treatment was 65, distributed as indicated: right orbicularis oculi 15U (3 punctures), left orbicularis oculi 15U (3 punctures), right corrugator 12,5U (1 puncture), left corrugator 12,5U (1 puncture), right frontalis 5U (1 puncture), and left frontalis 5U (1 puncture). The summary of the dilutions per patient and total Units per muscle and treatment are shown on tables 1-2. The treatment pattern is shown in Figure 1.

Table 1. Summary of patients and dilutions applied

Patients	Dilutions (ml)
Patient 1	0,5 vs 1
Patient 2	1 vs 0,25
Patient 3	0,25 vs1,5
Patient 4	1,5 vs 0,25
Patient 5	0,25 vs 0,5

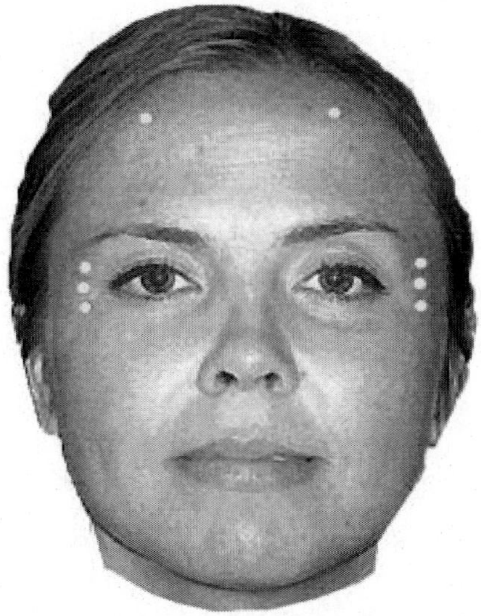

Figure 1. Treatment pattern. Ten total injection points divided in: RO (3points), LO (3points), RC (1point), LC (1point), RF (1point), LF (1point). RO: right orbicularis oculi muscle, LO: left orbicularis oculi muscle, RC: right corrugator muscle, LC: left corrugator muscle, RF: right frontalis muscle, LF: left frontalis muscle.

Table 2. Total units injected per muscle and treatment. R: right, L: left

Muscle	**Speywood Units**	**Punctures per Muscle**
R Orbicularis Oculi	15	3
L Orbicularis Oculi	15	3
R Corrugator	12,5	1
L Corrugator	12,5	1
R Frontalis	5	1
L Frontalis	5	1
Total	65	10

New Concepts

Before analyzing the results of the differential treatments we will introduce some new concepts.

- Minimal Responsive Dose (MRD):
  Corresponds to the minimum amount of toxin Units that generates a clinical effect, in a particular muscular area. If one is below this dose, no clinical benefit will be appreciable. It is specific of each target muscle and individual and may change in time.
- Maximum blockage Dose (MBD):
  It is defined as the amount of toxin Units that generates a maximal muscular clinical blockage, above which greater doses are not correlated with greater effect. It is specific of each target muscle and individual and may change in time.

The space between MRD and MBD is defined as *botulinum toxin therapeutic window (BTTW), and* is the area were clinical responses are variable and may be measured or evaluated. Outside of this area responses may be non-apparent or maximal, being extremely difficult to determine clinically any differences regarding drug dose or potency.

All above are novel terms and the exact values for general population are not yet been established.

Clinical Cases

- PATIENT 1. **0, 5 vs 1ml**

  This case shows a slightly higher right eyebrow before the treatment on the frontal view (Figures 2-3). After the treatment the eyebrow are symmetric showing a higher action on the right orbicularis oculi that allows ipsilateral frontal muscle to raise the brow. This event is verified in the more concentrated side.

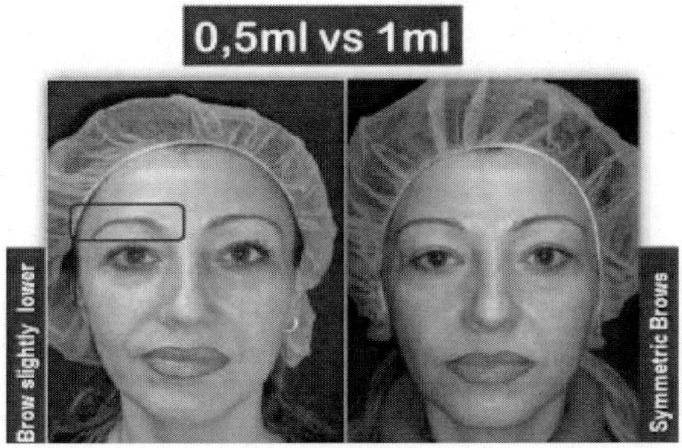

Figures 2-3. Patient 1. Frontal view before and after the treatment.

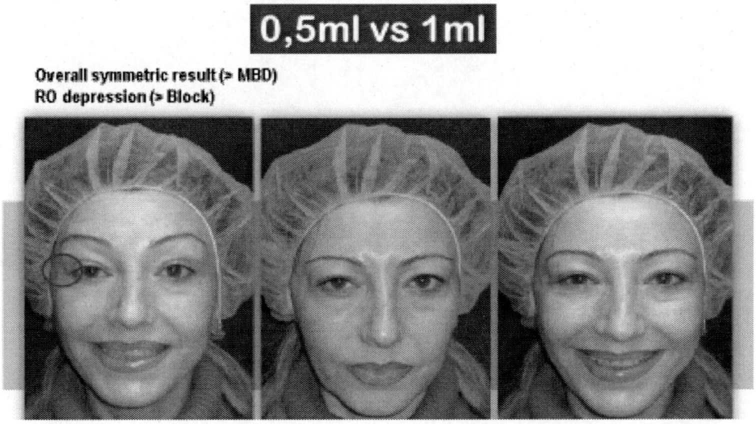

Figures 4-6. Patient 1. Analysis of facial motility after the treatment. Red circle highlights enhanced block action on the toxin concentrated side. MBD: maximal blockade dose. RO: right orbicularis oculi.

When analyzing the case on muscular action we observe an overall symmetric result. Probably in this case the maximal blockade dose was overlapped. Nevertheless a slight depression is seen on the right orbicularis oculi, showing a greater block on this side, ipsilateral to the more concentrated toxin side (Figures 4-6).

- Patient 2. **1 vs 0, 25 ml**

  This case shows a higher right eyebrow on the pretreatment frontal picture. After the treatment a more symmetric brow height is achieved. The left brow experimented a higher raising effect due to a more important block of the left orbicularis oculi, ipsilateral to the higher toxin concentration (figures 7-8).

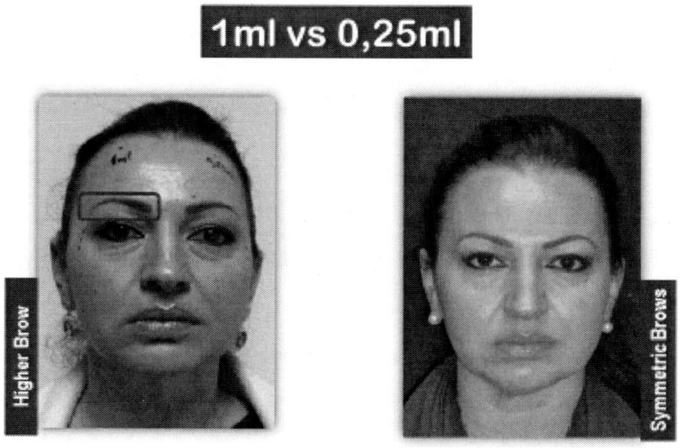

Figures 7-8. Patient 2. Frontal view pre and post treatment. Red rectangle shows higher right brow pretreatment.

When analyzing the case after treatment on muscular action we observe a more important frontal wrinkling on the more diluted right side. The glabellar area shows a left wrinkling deviation demonstrating a more important contractile strength on the right side (diluted). The right orbicularis oculi (diluted side) presents greater wrinkling (Figures 9-11).

- Patient 3. **0, 25 vs 1,5ml**

  This case shows a higher eyebrow on the left side prior to the toxin inoculation. The difference is smaller after the treatment, due to a more important right orbicularis oculi block and right brow raising (concentrated side). After treatment an area of depression is perceived on the right orbicularis oculi, associated with a higher block on the concentrated side (Figures 12-15).

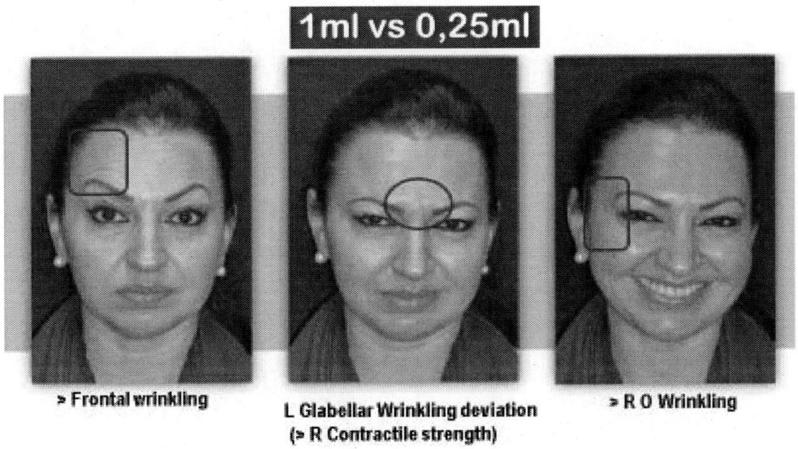

Figures 9-11. Patient 2. Post treatment facial motility analysis. Red figures sign differences. R: right; L: left; RO: right orbicularis oculi.

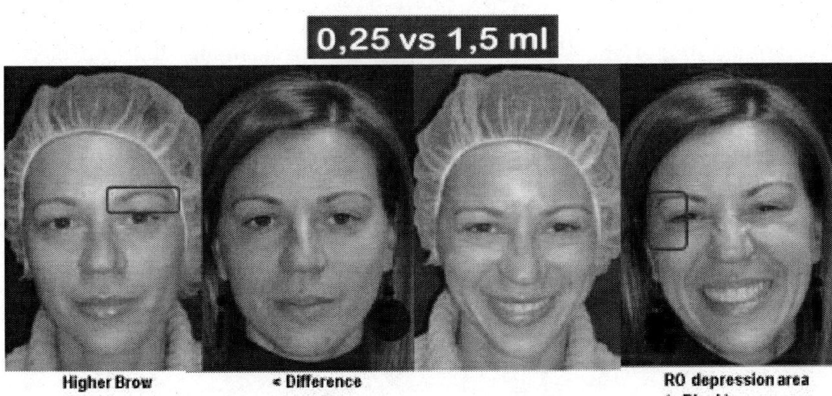

Figures 12-15. Patient 3. Frontal view at rest and smiling before and after treatment. Red rectangles highlight differences. RO: right orbicularis oculi.

Motility analysis reveals symmetric glabellar wrinkling before and after toxin inoculation. Probably maximal blockage dose was achieved bilaterally. Frontal wrinkling is superior on the diluted as marked on the red rectangle (Figures 16-19).

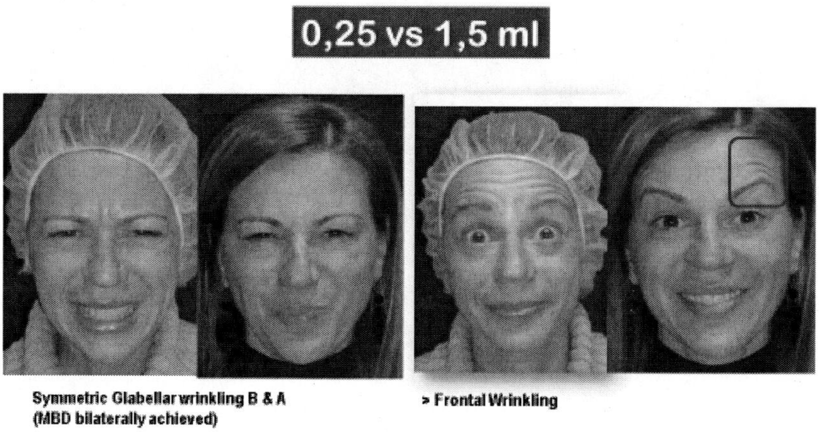

Figures 16-19. Patient 3. Facial motility differences pre and post treatment. Red rectangle shows more frontal wrinkling on the diluted side. MBD: maximal blockade dose, B: before, A: after.

Another important detail is the volume related to this differential treatments which cause greater discomfort, swelling and tissue distortion, immediately after the treatments (Figure 20).

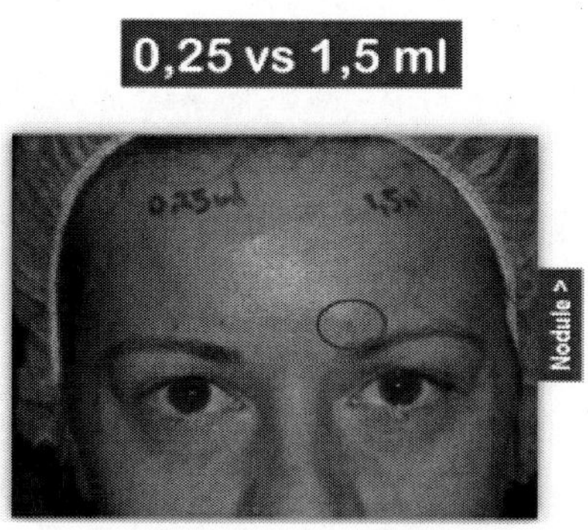

Figure 20. Patient 3. Detail of the immediate result after botulinum toxin injection. The difference on the nodule size is highlighted on the red oval.

- Patient 4. **1,5 vs 0,25ml**

This patient showed a lower left brow before treatment. After toxin injection the left brow (concentrated side) was higher than contralateral (Figures 21-24). The patient perceived this irregularity and further retouch was necessary to achieve symmetry.

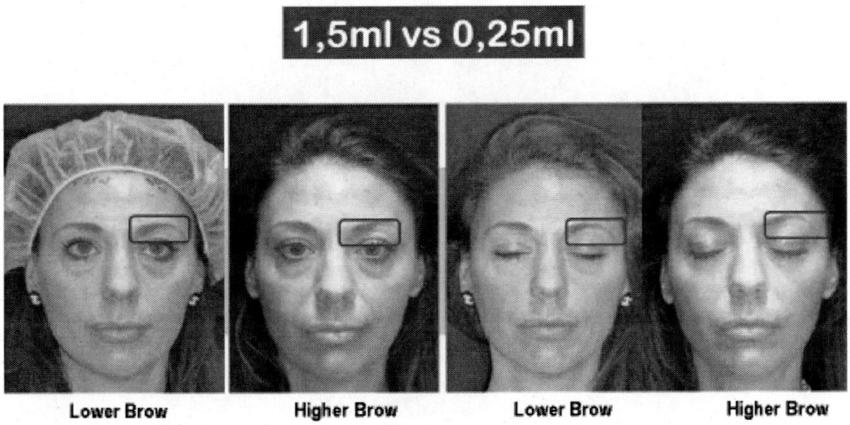

Figures 21-24. Patient 4. Frontal view at rest before and after toxin treatment. Red rectangles indicate effect on concentrated side.

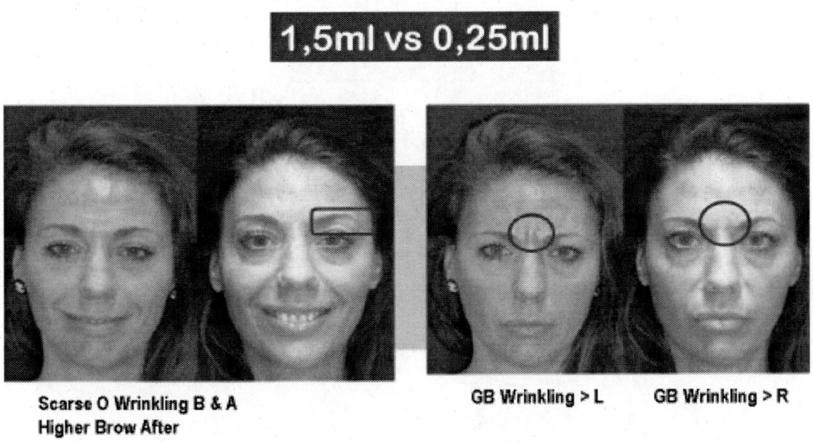

Figures 25-28. Patient 4. Facial motility analysis. Asymmetries are evidenced on red symbols. O: Orbicularis oculi, B: Before, A: After, GB: Glabella, L: Left, R: Right.

When analyzing facial motility, scarce wrinkling is perceived before and after the treatment on the orbicularis oculi portion. The glabella presents basally greater wrinkling on the left side. After treatment greater wrinkling is observed on the right diluted side (Figures 25-28).

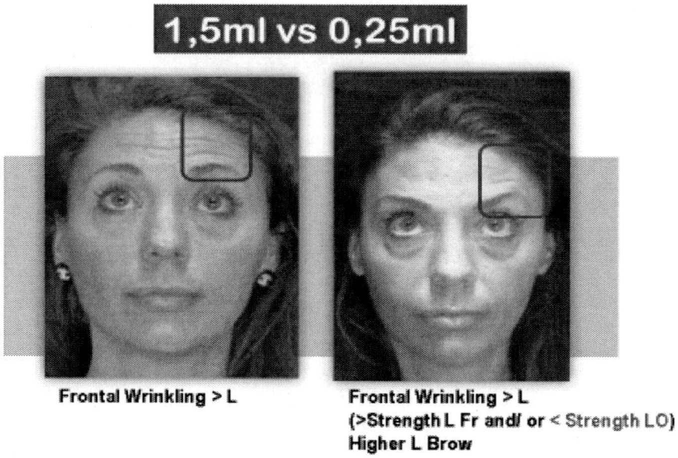

Figures 29-30. Patient 4. Frontal wrinkling. Asymmetries are highlight in red rectangles. L: left, LFr: left Frontalis Muscle, LO: left orbicularis.

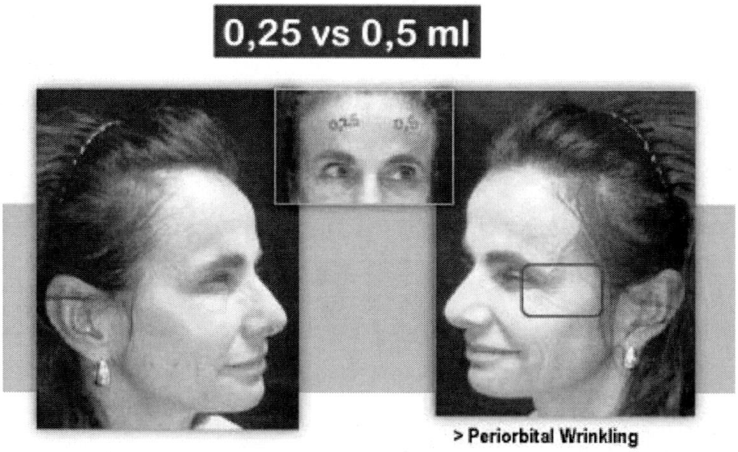

Figures 31-33. Patient 5. Differences on crow's feet wrinkles are evidenced in red rectangle.

Frontal activity is greater before and after treatment on the left side. Possible explanations are stronger left frontalis muscle or weaker left orbicularis oculi on the concentrated side that determines a higher left eyebrow (Figures 29-30).

- Patient 5. **0, 25 vs 0,5 ml**

  This patient experimented important asymmetry on the crow's feet area after toxin injection with more wrinkling (less drug action) on the diluted side (Figures 31-33). Further treatment was necessary to solve this condition.

Discussion

According to *Wikitionary* the term *Dilution* stands for a solution that has additional solvent, such as water, added to it into order to make it less concentrated. In chemistry, concentration is the abundance of a constituent divided by the total volume of a mixture. The term can be applied to any kind of chemical mixture, but most frequently it refers to solutes and solvents in solutions.

In this particular case, *dilution* is itself an inaccurate term, as *reconstitution* better describes combining solid prepackaged toxin with fluid. Among the substances that have been used to reconstitute botulinum toxin are normal saline, normal saline with the preservative benzyl alcohol, and lidocaine. The last two have been shown to markedly diminish injection pain without notable loss of effectiveness.

An open debate still prevails regarding the dissociation moment of the complex toxin- structural proteins, which is supposed to naturally occur at PH 7, 2. This is achieve in the body for some and for others is manifested within the vial after reconstitution. It has been proposed that by altering PH within the vial through different solvents, it may be enhance drug availability and action. Nevertheless, the former has not been scientifically supported.

Another important variable that may affect toxin efficacy is concentration, with fluid volumes of 1 to 10ml routinely used to reconstitute an entire vial of botulinum toxin.

According to the findings of the differential treatments, reduced volumes are associated with higher muscular blockage intensity. Higher toxin concentrations are related with higher drug potency and greater clinical benefits (block intensity and duration). This situation is appreciable within some limits, as which when Maximal Blockade Dose has been achieved, dilutions differences become irrelevant. As previously explained whenever the patient falls outside of BTTW clinical analysis is not useful. Moreover the lesser the injected volume, the minor the patient discomfort during the treatments and swelling post procedure.

Toxin diffusion has been a major concern since botulinum toxin FDA clearance for cosmetic purposes. Based on this findings and empirical experience, the author has developed a diffusion theory. This principle identifies 2 possible diffusions; micro diffusion and macro diffusion.

Micro diffusion is characteristic of each commercial product available and non-modifiable. It is determined by the toxin complex and the independent protein fraction in the form of human albumin. The less the albumin content the greater the micro diffusion will be. This type of dispersion is desirable and important, since it determines a more global muscular block, and a greater clinical effect and lasting. Micro dispersion allows the drug to affect more neuromuscular junctions and to obtain further significant benefits. The effect can be compared to augmenting the traction vectors to lift the affected tissue, when performing a face lift. This is a brand new concept, not described or published before. According to this, the intrinsic potency, intended as blocking action and lasting, of the different formulations available would be greater for abobotulinum, intermediate for onabotulinum and lesser for incobotulinum toxin A, being the latter the product with higher albumin content and minor micro diffusion. To modify this condition is that the manufacturers have established different volumes recommendations for reconstitution.

On the other hand, Macro diffusion is principally related to the reconstitution (dilution) volume used. It is a modifiable factor and seems to affect drug potency, and be associated with increased risk of complications, such as palpebral ptosis. Highly diluted toxins are linked to higher incidences of this event, due to an uncontrolled dispersion of the solvent (saline for the majority), that gets displaced from the *Corrugator* area to the *Levator Palpebrae Superioris* muscle. This concept was classically accepted as diffusion and attacked by media and related companies. On the contrary, the higher the toxin concentration, the safer the treatment will be and the lower the incidence of palpebral ptosis. The author has performed more than 7000 botulinum toxin treatments with 2 cases of palpebral ptosis documented, (way below standard incidence described as 1-3%), mainly explained by correct technique and highly concentrated toxin therapies. A summary on Torres

Diffusion theory is given on table 3. Recent appearance of dose clicker system syringes allows physicians to perform concentrated treatments precisely.

Table 3. Torres Toxin Diffusion Theory Summary

Micro Diffusion	Macro Diffusion
Albumin Related	Volume Related
Non Modifiable	Modifiable
Desirable	Non desirable
Associated with intrinsic drug potency	Associated with higher incidence of palpebral ptosis

By augmenting reconstitution volume, one can expect to reduce potency, affect a greater area by macro dispersion and compensate a scarse micro dispersion inherent of the product. This unfortunately will carry an increased risk of complications, as solvent dispersion is not really controllable.

Facial asymmetries are very common in normal population. Nonetheless, minimal asymmetries are not evidenced by the patients and unless careful exam, are neither perceived by physicians. However it is very important to analyze and document preexistent alterations. After toxin treatments the patient may start noticing some differences and may blame the new treatment as principal source of this unpleasant condition.

There are several variables that may affect botulinum toxin treatments effectivity, such as dilution, solvent use, dose, formulation, muscle group injected, depth of injection and force and speed of injection. All above indicate that treatment outcome is a much more complex process than previously expected. The understanding and mastery of all above will allow us to give better and more reliable treatments in the future.

References

Alam M. Practice gaps. Dilution, reconstitution, and complexity: comment on "A small study of the relationship between abobotulinum toxin A concentration and forehead wrinkle reduction." *Arch Dermatol.* 2012 Jan;148(1):119-21.

Anagnostou E, Rentzos M, Alexakis T, et al. Volume matters: the influence of different botulinum toxin-A dilutions for sialorrhea in amyotrophic lateral sclerosis. *Muscle Nerve.* 2013 Feb;47(2):276-8. doi: 10.1002/mus.23692. Epub 2012 Dec 28.

Arch Dermatol. 2012 Jan;148(1):121-2. doi: 10.1001/ archderm. 148.1.121.

Boyle MH, McGwin G Jr, Flanagan CE, et al. High versus low concentration botulinum toxin A for benign essential blepharospasm: does dilution make a difference? *Ophthal Plast Reconstr Surg.* 2009 Mar-Apr;25(2):81-4. doi:10.1097/IOP.0b013e31819946c4.

Brodsky MA, Swope DM, Grimes D. Diffusion of botulinum toxins. *Tremor Other Hyperkinet Mov.* 2012;2. pii: tre-02-85-417-1. Epub 2012 Aug 6.

Eisele KH, Fink K, Vey M, et al. Studies on the dissociation of botulinum neurotoxin type A complexes. *Toxicon.* 2011 Mar 15;57(4):555-65. doi: 10.1016/j.toxicon.2010.12.019. Epub 2010 Dec 30.

Gracies JM, Lugassy M, Weisz DJ, et al. Botulinum toxin dilution and endplate targeting in spasticity: a double-blind controlled study. *Arch Phys Med Rehabil.* 2009 Jan;90(1):9-16.e2. doi: 10.1016/ j.apmr.2008.04.030.

Güleç AT. Dilution of botulinum toxin A in lidocaine vs. in normal saline for the treatment of primary axillary hyperhidrosis: a double-blind, randomized, comparative preliminary study. *J Eur Acad Dermatol Venereol.* 2012 Mar;26(3):314-8. doi:10.1111/j.1468-3083.2011.04066.x. Epub 2011 Apr 15.

Kim A, Jung J, Pak A. Botulinum toxin type A reconstituted in lidocaine with epinephrine for facial rejuvenation:results of a participant satisfaction survey.*Cutis* 2013 Jul;Suppl:13-8.

Ramirez-Castaneda J, Jankovic J, Comella C, et al. Diffusion, spread, and migration of botulinum toxin. *Mov Disord.* 2013 Nov;28(13):1775-83. doi: 10.1002/mds.25582. Epub 2013 Jul 18.

Trindade De Almeida AR, Secco LC, Carruthers A. Handling botulinum toxins: an updated literature review. *Dermatol Surg* 2011 Nov;37(11):1553-65. doi: 10.1111/j.1524 -4725.2011.02087.x.Epub 2011 Jul 21.

In: Botulinum Toxins and Botulism
Editor: Charlotte Reynolds
ISBN: 978-1-63483-384-4

Chapter 5

Botulism Type E from Native Foods in the Arctic Regions

***B. Zane Horowitz*[1] *and Keahi Mookini Horowitz*[2]**
[1]Oregon-Alaska Poison Center, Oregon Health and Science University, US
[2]John A. Burns School of Medicine, University of Hawaii, US

Abstract

Botulism in the Arctic regions has occurred with some unique food sources. Native fermentation of fish heads, fish eggs, and beaver tail allow proper conditions for botulinum toxin to be elaborated from *Clostridium botulinum*. The consumption of whale meat with the skin attached (*muktuk*) also had been associated with outbreaks of botulism. These unique foods are not consumed anywhere else in the world, and have a disproportionate association with botulism clusters. Cases of botulism from consuming these foods in Alaska and Canada have been described for more than a century. The serotype implicated in botulism from native Arctic foods is almost always type E. Coastal soils from this part of the world are rich in botulism type E. The other distinguishing characteristics of type E botulism is that it can withstand freezing down to 3.5 ^{o} Celsius, and that it is not saccharolytic, unlike types A and B. Type E botulism has been associated with Norwegian "rakfisk" preparation, a process similar to fermented Arctic foods. Importation of vacuum-packed whitefish from Alaska and Canada has also been associated with sporadic cases of botulism in Europe.

Introduction

Subsistence fishing and hunting in the arctic regions of the world has sustained a small but constant population of circumpolar indigenous peoples. Their food choices have been ones of necessity. Contrary to its perception, the arctic abounds in fish and game, but these often must be stored for times when hunting is not successful. To survive the winters the circumpolar peoples have developed a variety of food preservation skills handed down through the generations. Unfortunately some of these food preservation techniques have fostered the growth of *Clostridium botulinum* that elaborates botulism toxin-type E.

The circumpolar peoples inhabit Alaska, Canada, Greenland, and parts of Scandinavia and Russia. Originating from the ancient Thule people, the Inuit migrated from the Bering Strait region of Northern Alaska between the years 1000 and 1600, moving island to island in small groups into what is now known as Arctic Canada and Greenland. They brought with them advanced hunting and fishing skills, allowing them to survive on larger ocean mammals such as whale, walrus, and seal [1]. The term Eskimo, although rarely used today, is broadly inclusive of the two major groups, the Yupik of Alaska and the Inuit (which includes the Kalaallit of Greenland, Inuit and Inuvialuit of Canada, and the Inupiat of Alaska). Yupik of Alaska still have counterparts today in eastern Siberia, and their common ancestors may have been the indigenous people who first crossed to North America across the Beringian land bridge from Russia to the Alaskan Arctic centuries ago. A separate group, the Aleuts, inhabit the 1900-kilometer long chain of Aleutian Islands in the southwest, and Kamchatka in Russia. In the interior of Northern Canada reside the Athabascans who inhabit western inland Canada from the Yukon westward into central Alaska. Although not within the Arctic Circle there are several important northwest Pacific coastal tribes in British Columbia, Haida Gwaii (formerly the Queen Charlotte Islands), and into southeast Alaska of which the Haida, Tlingit, and Tsimshian are the largest. Some of these Pacific coast First Nation tribes have also been the source of Native food occurrences of botulism [2]. Siberian Yupik, Chukchi in Russia, and the Sami people (previously known as Lapps or Laplanders) in Scandinavia are the other circumpolar peoples, but there is no published information characterizing the occurrences of botulism among them.

Accurate descriptions of arctic botulism in the medical literature in Canada date back to 1919 [3, 4]. Some have speculated that botulism has been responsible for earlier clusters of deaths in the Arctic in both native peoples and possibly European explorers [4]. The medical papers of Claude Ernest Dolman, describe in detail many of these early Canadian outbreaks [3, 4, 5, 6]. Dolman continued to document botulism occurrences in the Canadian Arctic for over 60 years. He first characterized these botulism occurrences correctly as type E botulinum toxin in 1944 in Nanaimo, British Columbia [5, 6]. Similarly since 1947 the medical literature has documented similar trends in coastal remote Alaskan communities [7]. From analysis of the available national databases it is clear that the incidence of botulism in this area is amongst the highest in the world. The population of Alaska comprises less than 0.2% of the United States but has as recently since 1990 been the site of 39% of all U.S. botulism cases, with 90% of these Alaskan occurrences being type E [2, 7].

Type E Botulism

Clostridium species have a natural habitat in the soils of the world. *Clostridium botulinum* may produce the serotype toxins A thru H. *Clostridium baratii* has also been implicated in Type E human disease [8]. Type E producing *Clostridium botulinum* is prevalent in the coastal arctic soils and in fish entrails [6]. Type E is not present in the coasts around the United Kingdom, but is found in Scandinavia and the Baltic [6]. Type E producing strains are more resistant to freezing down to 3.5^{o} Celsius than types A and B [8].

Under stress the dormant organism *Clostridium botulinum* forms a spore that can survive low heat cooking and certain food preservation techniques. Type E toxin, by its natural resistance to lower temperatures, may start germination under thawing and partial re-freezing [6]. Germination is essential to elaborate the toxin, and in most cases of food-borne botulism toxin elaboration has occurred prior to ingestion of the food when the food has been improperly handled, preserved and prepared [2, 9]. If food is stored in a moist environment with anaerobic conditions, low acidity ($pH < 4.5$), and low salinity, the botulinum spore can germinate. Inadvertent consumption of these products will lead to the classic food associated botulism. However, two groups of individuals may develop disease from ingestion of spores rather than preformed toxin. In both young infants, and adults with prior complex gastrointestinal surgery and gastrointestinal motility dysfunction, conditions in their intestines allow for ingested spores to germinate.

Serotype A and B producing Clostridium are more likely to be saccharolytic, fermenting foods to short chained fatty acids and at times may cause an unpleasant bitter odor or taste in the food. Type E is not saccharolytic and no change in odor or taste occurs, although traditional native food preparation techniques impart a strong odor to their fermented foods [10].

Alaska

The types of food eaten and prepared by Natives in the Alaskan arctic are from animals and fish that are prevalent in the area. This subsistence hunting and fishing has served them well over time but certain preparation rituals have now been understood to foster the development of botulism.

A unique preparation method of fermenting or putrefying foods is common in Alaska, and has been part of the traditional Inuit diet for centuries. These "stink" foods are "Stink Heads" made from salmon heads or "Stink Eggs" made from salmon eggs [2, 6, 11]. Originally salmon heads, salmon eggs, seal meat, or whale blubber, was placed in an animal-skin lined pit and covered with moss and allowed to ferment for several weeks. This process first described by Nelson in the 1880's indicated that the summer catch of salmon have the heads cut off, placed in pits surrounded by turf and straw and left until the bones have decayed to a gelatinous mass [2]. Also called "tipmuk" salmon it may be putrefied in a willow leaf lined pit and left to decay for a month or more [4, 6] [Figure 1].

The "stink eggs" are putrefied similarly in lined pits and are allowed to reach a state of mass resembling cheese, with a firm outer surface but soft center [2]. This practice of making "stink eggs" is prevalent along the southern Alaska and British Columbia's Pacific coast. Some modifications of this technique includes covering the food in seal oil, which often serves unknowingly to promote anaerobic conditions. Since salmon is mostly caught in the summer, these "stink head" and "stink egg" outbreaks tend to occur in late summer or the fall [15]. Seal skins have also been used as the container for fermentation and sometimes the skins are hung up in the residence instead of being buried, allowing exposure to higher temperatures, therefore providing an optimal environment for spore germination [6]. As outside influences impinged on the Inuit each technologic advance unfortunately only served to promote better anaerobic germinating conditions. The use of small barrels instead of animal skins began around the 1940's and this allowed easier burial and retrieval, and sometimes these were left in the sun or indoors [2, 12, 13]. Barrels though seemingly cleaner than using animal skins, can be sealed tighter and promote anaerobic conditions. In more recent years the use of plastic lids on barrels, glass Mason jars, sealable plastic bags, and sealed plastic containers have all improved hygienic conditions but have allowed anaerobic conditions needed for botulism toxin to thrive [14, 15, 16, 17]. Even when Native Alaskans move from their family villages to larger population centers they sometimes continue to prepare their native foods, and use of common kitchen sealable plastic containers have been associated with an increase in botulism occurrence [15].

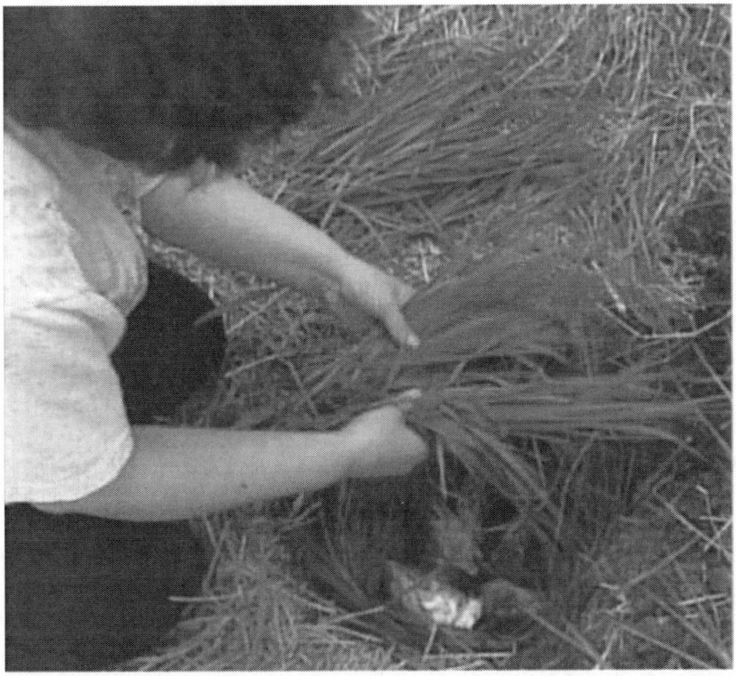

Figure 1. The Making of "Tipmuk," or "Stinky head" process. Salmon heads are buried in a shallow pit covered by willow leaves and left to ferment for several weeks to months.(Photo public domain: from Center for Disease Control and Prevention, and the Arctic Investigations Program).

Mammalian meat has been associated with a few cases; especially seal meat, beaver tail ("stinky tail"), or dried beaver paw. Most of these have been due to improper storage of these meats [2]. Several outbreaks occurred amongst the Yupik natives in the western area of Alaska surrounding Bristol Bay [15, 16, 17]. The Yupik have the highest occurrence of botulism due to their traditional preparation methods, whereas the Aleuts and Athabascans rarely have been cited in outbreaks of botulism from Native foods [15]. The beaver run typically occurs in the spring, and botulism outbreaks occur in summer and fall. In one outbreak in Bristol Bay Alaska the food preparer wrapped fresh beaver tail in plastic and left if near the stove for 2 weeks before she and two other women ate it. Two of the women died within 24 hours from the onset of symptoms [15]. In another outbreak in the city of Dillingham beaver tails were fermented, then frozen for several months. They were first placed in a barrel covered with moss and water, then allowed to dry for 2 weeks before the "stinky tail" was consumed. Seven of 15 people who consumed this developed botulism. Interestingly 3 cases were confirmed as type B [15]. In another occurrence seal flippers were left in a bucket covered with moss for 5 days inside in warm environment before it was consumed and caused a non-fatal case of botulism. One food preparer interviewed during an epidemiologic investigation of an outbreak expressed concern that as a child she learned of superstition of the "Killing Rays of the Sun" and knew she was not supposed to leave these barrels outside above ground [15].

One unique food associated with botulism in the North American Arctic includes "muktuk," an Inuit delicacy made from whale blubber with the skin attached. Numerous cases of botulism associated with "muktuk" in both Alaska and the Canadian Arctic have been documented since the 1950's, but its association with outbreaks still persists today [6, 12].

In one outbreak in 1959 a boating party of Inuit ate portions of a decaying beached whale; 7 of 8 natives who ingested the fluke developed botulism within 24 hours, all but one recovered [4]. Specimens obtained confirmed Type E botulism at autopsy. In a nearly exact scenario in July 2002 a beached Beluga whale was found in Kwigillinggok, a remote village in western Alaska on the Bering Strait, and it was likely dead for sometime [18]. The villagers did not believe however that it had decayed and "muktuk" was cut from the tail and stored in sealable plastic bags, and subsequently consumed. Of the 14 villagers who consumed "muktuk" eight villagers developed botulism over the next 3 days. This was confirmed as type E botulism in one patient, and from the "muktuk" specimens, by the Center for Disease Control (CDC) [18].

In Alaska, a monovalent type E antitoxin had been available from Canada, and was used along with the bivalent FDA approved antitoxin with an Investigational New Drug protocol in Alaska until 2010, when both antitoxins were retired in favor of the heptavalent antitoxin now in use. However the type E antitoxin was rarely used by itself. It was originally manufactured at the University of Toronto by Connaught Medical Research Labs, and used experimentally in Hokkaido, Japan. On Hokkaido, the Northern-most island of Japan, where "izushi" is a traditional food. This fish is fermented and preserved in rice. Twenty-one outbreaks associated with "izushi" were reported between 1951 and 1965. There were 138 cases of botulism, where 40 patients died. All were type E botulism [19]. The Canadian antitoxin for type E was not used in these early outbreaks as it did not become available until 1959. The case fatality ratio after type E antitoxin was instituted in Japan fell from 29% prior to the availability of the type E antitoxin, to 3.5% in 85 patients treated with the type E antitoxin. Shortly after the initial success of the Canadian antitoxin in Japan, the Japanese National Institute of Health created their own type E antitoxin [19].

Canada

There appear to be two separate geographic areas where most Canadian botulism outbreaks have occurred, each associated with a different native food. In the Arctic North, in current Nunavut Territory (which encompasses the Canadian Arctic Archipelago and Baffin Island), Northwest Territories, Nunavik in northern Quebec, and Labrador botulism cases have been associated with traditional Inuit foods [3, 6, 20, 21]. Fermented seal meat, known as "utjak," was responsible for ten occurrences in Labrador between 1956 and 1962, along a 240 kilometer sparsely inhabited east Labrador coastline [3, 20]. "Utjak" is made of uncooked seal flippers preserved in seal oil, and allowed to acquire its taste through fermentation. This is usually kept indoors in a barrel, often near the stove, providing warm temperatures necessary for botulinum toxin to develop from spores. One case report showed the disadaptation of technology, in that the "utjak" was fermented in an abandoned oil drum [22]. Oral tradition, cited by Dolman, speaks of whole families who died from bad seal meat, going back several generations [4]. One case in Labrador was traced to raw seal liver eaten from a decaying carcass stored under the porch for a month [4].

One of the earliest documented type E cases occurred in 1932, and involved salmon from Labrador that was imported to Cooperstown, NY [6]. Originally attributed to a new type of Clostridium, it was later characterized as type E. The first trials of the Canadian Connaught Medical Research Laboratories type E antitoxin were conducted in Labrador in 1960, before being used in the outbreak in Japan [4]. Between 1945 and 1969 Baffin Island Inuit had 19 cases of botulism in 4 local outbreaks from seal meat, with 14 afflicted individuals dying [3]. Only one individual was able to receive antitoxin, and she survived. Harp Seal, or "kairulik," caught in June, stored and eaten in September, was responsible for 10 cases of botulism on Baffin Island in 1969 [20]. Seven patients in this outbreak received trivalent antitoxin and all survived, while the three patients who could not receive antitoxin died [19]. Seven additional outbreaks in Nunavut (then Northern Quebec) occurred between 1964 and 1975, with 25 Inuit affected, eight of whom died [3]. One of these cases involved fermented walrus meat or "igunaq." One outbreak involving 11 Inuit was from consuming sun-dried beluga whale [3]. Ten of these Inuit in this outbreak who received trivalent antitoxin survived. Two outbreaks involving seal flippers occurred in the Northwest Territories, one of which the seal flipper was stored in a plastic bag and kept near the stove [3].

The Pacific coast of British Columbia represents the second area of local botulism activity. The indigenous First Nations tribes in the Pacific include the Haida, Tlingit, and Tsimshian. Here the food implicated in botulism outbreaks was salmon eggs in all cases [3, 4]. There were 18 outbreaks, with 42 individual botulism cases, of which 11 died. Some of these outbreaks were traced to the "Stink Egg" preparation method also seen in the Alaskan outbreaks [3, 4, 21]. One case occurred in Whitehorse in the Yukon Territory in 1940 in a variation on this technique the fish eggs were fermented in a moose bladder for ten days [4]. Twenty-four cases were treated with some formulation of antitoxin and all of these cases survived. The death rate was 65% in 17 other cases who did not receive antitoxin [4].

Arctic Explorers

Almost certainly circumpolar native peoples died from botulism food poisoning for many centuries. Early accounts by arctic whalers of "ptomaine poisoning" may have been botulism [3, 6]. In her biography of Alaskan Native Ada Blackjack, Jennifer Niven mentions the death of Ada's father in Spruce

Creek, Alaska in 1906 after eating "meat that was too old" [23]. Did the Europeans who ventured into this unfamiliar environment also die from botulism? Vilhjalmur Stefansson's 1906 -1907 exploration of the Canadian Mackenzie River delta, , brought the first accounts published in 1914 of clusters of deaths, including eight who died eating a freshly caught whale that Dolman has ascribed to botulism [6].

The greatest number of deaths during the era of European exploration occurred in during a single expedition to the Arctic. The Franklin expedition set out from England with two ships, the *Eerebus* and *Terror*, in 1845 in an attempt to find the long-sought Northwest Passage across the Arctic and got stuck in the ice near King William Island in what is today part of the Nunavut Territory of Northern Canada. Over the first winter 3 sailors died and were buried with grave markers on Beechey Island [24, 25]. Over the next winter 18 more had died, including John Franklin himself. Given that they were well provisioned for 3 years, deaths at sea of this proportion and mostly of officers, was unheard of in the English Admiralty. Eventually the remaining 105 survivors tried to walk out of the arctic and died in groups along the way likely from starvation and scurvy [24, 26]. Over a century after the discovery of the Beechey Island graves, the bodies from the 3 graves from the first winter's casualties were exhumed in 1984. They had been preserved nearly completely intact by the permafrost [25, 26].

In his book Frozen in Time, Dr. Owen Beattie describes the project to exhume these bodies and conduct autopsies on them. He mentions one detail from the autopsy analysis of one of the sailor's intestine; it harbored an unspecified species of Clostridium [25]. Scott Cookman, in his book Iceblink, first argued that the Clostridium was botulism from the hastily provisioned tinned meat ordered by Franklin from the provider Goldners in England [26]. Dr. Beattie favored the argument that the tinned meat contained high levels of lead that may have killed the 3 sailors he exhumed in 1984 [25]. In fact lead exposure was pervasive in Victorian England, but rarely fatal in adults. Botulism, however, was unheard of in England, and despite Goldners provisioning of many other voyages, no other cases of botulism occurred [25]. An alternative explanation has since been argued that botulism may have been acquired by the efforts of the Franklin expedition experienced ice explorers in their efforts to acquire food [24]. Francis Crozier, Franklin's second in command was a seasoned arctic traveler [27]. Perhaps he, and others ate indigenous game, in an attempt to adapt native practices to survive the iced-bound winters. Small clusters of deaths from type E botulism is characteristic of Arctic botulism, with the fresh thawed game more likely going disproportionately to the ranks of the officers who died in greater numbers than the seaman [24]. Whatever speculation based on this single autopsy on the subject of the causation of deaths in the Franklin expedition, clearly botulism was not responsible for all the deaths of the 129 men on the Franklin expedition.

Franklin's submerged ship, the *Erebus,* has been recently located in the Canadian Arctic and perhaps recovery of human remains within may provide new clues to the greatest English naval disaster in the age of exploration.

Dr. Mark Personne, the medical director of the Stockholm Poison Center, has put forth a similar theory about the fate of the 1897 Swedish Andree expedition [28]. Three balloonists attempted to cross the North Pole from Sweden but their balloon crashed two days into the expedition. They survived from July until October on the ice and left an extensive diary of their ordeal up to their deaths.

The diary, undeveloped film, and the remains of the three explorers were found in 1930 on White Island, Svalbard.

Personne speculates that based on the diary evidence of consumption of seal meat, previously implicated in Canadian occurrences of botulism, and the sudden last entry on Oct 17, 1897 without notes of starvation, that botulism from the seal meat could have been the cause of a sudden death in the three Andree balloonists [28].

North Atlantic

In eastern Greenland in 1993, type E botulism was traced to a meal of seal meat and seal intestines [29]. Four of 8 participants in this meal developed clinical signs of botulism, two of which required ventilator assistance. The authors speculate that historically botulism was likely a problem in Greenland [29]. Type E botulism clusters continue to occur there. Seven cases of botulism have been reported on the Faroe Islands from eating dried mutton, one was type E [30].

Scandinavia

There are no cases of botulism from Arctic indigenous food in Scandinavian nations reported in the medical literature. Denmark reported 32 cases of botulism between 1901 and 1958 [4, 6]. Implicated foods included salted or pickled mackerel, herring, and liver loaf. A few cases of local fish related botulism prepared according to Norwegian custom, which bear some similarity to Inuit preparation practices, have been reported [31]. A case of char porridge, an arctic fish related to trout, has been linked retrospectively to botulism in 1831 in Osterdalen, Norway [32]. Since 1975 there have been 22 cases of type E botulism in Norway attributed to half-fermented "rakfisk." "Rakfisk" by home preparation is popular around Christmas [33]. The fish is prepared by adding salt (6% to 8% of the weight of the fish) and sugar to the gutted fish, which is then put into a pot under pressure. The pot is stored in a cool place (5–8ºC) and eaten without cooking after two to three months. In one such family outbreak, the fish was first fermented in a cellar at 13°C for three weeks, and only then refrigerated at 7°C. This preparation method for fish may have provided an excellent anaerobic medium for Clostridium to germinate at above freezing temperatures. This preparation method bears some similarity to barrel preparation of fish in Alaska, which replaced traditional methods.

Several Russian language articles attest to the presence of botulism in Russia, including type E associated with eating fish [34, 35, 36]. In 1934 and 1935 the first occurrences associated with fish were noted [3, 6]. These cases were unable to be neutralized by antitoxin against serotypes A and B, raising the likelihood that they represented type E botulism [6]. Smoked herring has been associated with type E botulism cases in Leningrad (1938) and pickled herring in an outbreak in Frederiksberg, Denmark (1951) [6]. Cases of type E botulism from smoked "kunzha," or salted fish were first reported in Kamchatka and on Sakhalin Island in the Russian north and far east, in the 1960s [35, 36].

Imported Arctic Seafood

Despite a paucity of botulism in the United Kingdom, there was an outbreak reported in 1979 in which four elderly individuals ate tinned salmon from Alaska [37]. More than a year had passed since the salmon was processed on Unimak Island, Alaska, and when it was purchased. Subsequent investigation found a small area of damage to the can. Two elderly couples in Birmingham took tea with salmon salad at 5 pm and by the next day all had vomiting, blurred vision, dry mouth, and ocular paralysis. Their symptoms progressed rapidly to near total paralysis, and all required intubation in less than 24 hours since the ingestion occurred. Within 4 hours of admission all were treated with the trivalent antitoxin, halting the progression of paralysis. Unfortunately, even though the antitoxin was given in less than 24 hours after ingestion, they all had an extended ICU courses with 2 of the patients dying on day 17 and day 23 post-exposure [37]. No other tins recalled from this batch canned in Alaska demonstrated botulism. Whitefish associated botulism had also been traced to an outbreak at a remote fish camp in Alaska in 1973 [38].

In 1982 a couple in Belgium ate canned salmon and developed botulism. One of them died and an international investigation and recall was begun [39]. The can was sold by a firm in Liverpool, England, but was obtained from a shipper in Seattle, Washington and a packing firm in Alaska. The can implicated was packed two years earlier, and similar lots from the same packinghouse had been distributed to Belgium, the Netherlands, and South Africa. A small hole was found in the can belonging to the index couple, and investigations showed 22 more dented and perforated cans found during a massive FDA mandated recall, from more than one Alaskan cannery. By the end of the investigation over 9 million dollars had been spent recalling 60 million cans of salmon from 314,000 food outlets; and stricter rules for can manufacturing and inspection were instituted in both the US and Canada [39].

In 1997 two Germans were diagnosed with botulism after eating imported hot-smoked Canadian whitefish, which was marketed in Finland [40]. The serum sample of one of the patients was identified as type E botulism. *Clostridium botulinum* was isolated from the fish sample and it was confirmed to be type E. The pulsed-field gel electrophoresis pattern of the isolated strain resembled a reference strain of North American origin, and did not match any *Clostridium botulinum* strains isolated from the Baltic Sea [40]. When Finnish trout farms were studied 10% of the samples were positive for botulism type E, but with proper food handling with high salinity and the addition of 0.1% sodium nitrate in the curing process the toxin could be eliminated [41]. Unfortunately another event occurred in Finland in 2006 also with a Canadian imported vacuum packed whitefish, which was associated with a case of type E botulism. An elderly woman ate the imported fish and developed progressive paralysis requiring ventilator assistance [42]. Imported Canadian whitefish continues to be an occasional cause of botulism type E in Europe, with a recent occurrence affecting 3 people in France in 2009 [43].

Conclusion

Type E botulism occurs in the arctic regions. Alaska fermented or "stink" preparation techniques has the highest association with botulism. Yupik technique of making "stinky tail" from fermented beaver tail has caused botulism. "Stinky heads" of salmon, or "tipmuk," are associated with botulism amongst the Yupik and Inuit. A similarly prepared fermented fish, "rakfisk," in Norway has been linked to type E botulism. Along the Pacific coast "Stink eggs" are associated with most cases of botulism. "Muktuk," a delicacy of whale blubber with the skin attached, and "Utjak," uncooked seal flippers in seal oil, are both Inuit foods from the Canadian Arctic and Alaska associated with botulism. Seal meat has been associated with botulism cases in Greenland and Canada. Of the future considerations for prevention of botulism in the Arctic would be the development of a type E toxoid vaccine, and a public health immunization program for Alaskan and Canadian Native peoples.

References

[1] Stern, P. R. & Stevenson, L. (2006). *Critical Inuit Studies: An Anthology of Contemporary Arctic Ethnography.* University of Nebraska Press, Lincoln, Nebraska.

[2] Castrodale, L. (2005). "Botulism in Alaska: A Guide for Physicians and Healthcare Providers: 2005 Update." Produced by the Department of Health and Social Services, Division of Public Health, Section of Epidemiology.

[3] Dolman, C. E. (1974). Human Botulism in Canada (1919-1973). *Canada Med Assoc Journal, 110*, 191-198.

[4] Dolman, C. E. (1961). Further Outbreaks of Botulism in Canada. *Canada Med Assoc Journal. 84,* 191-200.

[5] Dolman, C.E., & Kerr, D. E. (1948). Two Fatal Cases of Botulism from Home-Bottled Asparagus. *Canada Med Assoc. Journal. 59*, 412-414.

[6] Dolman, C. (1960). Type E Botulism: A Hazard of the North. *Arctic*, *13*, 230-256.

[7] Sobel, J., Tucker, N., Sulka, A., McLaughlin, J., & Maslanka, S. (2004). Foodborne Botulism in the United States, 1990-2000. *Emerging Infectious Diseases, 10*, 1606-1611.

[8] Horowitz, B. Z. (2005), Botulinum Toxin, *Critical Care Medicine, 21(4),*825-839.

[9] Sobel J, (2005), Botulism, *Clinical Infectious Disease*, *41*,1167 -1177.

[10] Gerwing, J, Dolman, C.E., & Arnott, D.A. (1961). Purification and Activation of *Clostridium Botulinum* Type E Toxin. *J Bacteriology*, *81*, 819-822.

[11] Castrodale, L., & Smith, B. (2006). Memorandum: Botulism Yukon-Kuskokwim Delta. State of Alaska Department of Health and Social Services Division of Public Health, Section of Epidemiology.

[12] Eisenberg, M.S, & Bender, T. R. (1976). Botulism in Alaska, 1947 Through 1974: Early Detection of Cases and Investigation of Outbreaks as a Means of Reducing Mortality. *Journal American Medical Association, 235*, 35-38.

[13] Wainwright, R. B., Heyward, W. L., Middaugh, J. P., Hatheway, C. L. Harpster, A. P., & Bender, T. R. (1988). Food-Borne Botulism in Alaska, 1947-1985: Epidemiology and Clinical Findings. *Journal of Infectious Diseases, 157*, 1158-1162.

[14] Barrett, D. H. (1991). Endemic Food-Borne Botulism: Clinical Experience, 1973-1986 at Alaska Native Medical Center. *Alaska Medicine, 33*, 101-108.

[15] Shaffer, N., Wainwright, R. B., Middaugh, J. P., & Tauxe, R. V. (1990). Botulism Among Alaska Natives: The Role of Changing Food Preparation and Consumption Practices. *Western Journal of Medicine, 153,* 390-393.

[16] Chiou, L.A., Hennessy, T.W. Hornhennessy, A., Horn, A.C., Butler, J.C., (2002) Botulism among Alaska natives in the Bristol Bay area of Southwest Alaska: A Survey of knowledge, attitudes, and practices related to fermented foods known to cause botulism, *International J Circumpolar Health, 61(1),* 50-60.

[17] Eisenberg, M.D. & Bender, T. R. (1976). Plastic Bags and Botulism: A New Twist To An Old Hazard of the North. *Alaska Medicine, 18*, 47-49.

[18] McLauglin, J. B., Sobel, J., Lynn, T., Funk, E., & Middaugh, J. P. (2004). Botulism Type E Outbreak Associated with Eating a Beached Whale, Alaska. *Emerging Infectious Diseases, 10*, 1685-1687.

[19] Nishiura, H. (2007). Incubation Period as a Clinical Predictor of Botulism: Analysis of Previous Izushi-Borne Outbreaks in Hokkaido, Japan, from 1951-1965. *Epidemiology. Infection, 135*, 126-130.

[20] Stuart, P. F., Wiebe, E. J., McElroy, R., Cameron, D. E., Todd, E. C. D., Erdman, I. E., Albalas, B., & Pivnick, H. (1970). Botulism Among Cape

Dorset Eskimos and Suspected Botulism at Frobisher Bay and Wakeham Bay. *Canadian Journal of Public Health, 61*, 509-517.

[21] Hauschild, A. H. W. & Gauvreau, L. (1985). Food-borne Botulism in Canada, 1971-84. *Canada Med Assoc Journal*, 133, 1141-1146.

[22] Brocklehurst, J.C. (1957). Medical Memorandum: Fatal Outbreak of Botulism Among Labrador Eskimos. *British Medical Journal, 924.*

[23] Niven J. (2003) *Ada Blackjack: A True Story of Survival in the Arctic.* Hyperion, NY.

[24] Horowitz, B.Z. (2003). Polar Poisons: Did Botulism Doom the Franklin Expedition?, *Journal of Toxicology, 41*, 841-847.

[25] Beattie, O. & Geiger, J. (1998). *Frozen in Time: The Fate of the Franklin Expedition*, Greystone, Vancouver, Canada.

[26] Cookman, S. (2000). *Iceblink: The Tragic Fate of Sir John Franklin's Lost Polar Expedition*, John Wiley & Sons, NY.

[27] Smith, M. (2006). *Captain John Crozier: Last Man Standing?,* Collins Press, Cork, Ireland.

[28] Personne, M. (2000). Andrée-expeditionens män dog troligen av botulism, *Lakartidningen, 97*, 12.

[29] Sorenen, H.C. (1993). Botulism in Ammassalik, *Ugeskr Laeger, 155(2)*,108-109.

[30] Wandall, E.P. & Videro, T. (1991). Botulism on the Faeroe Islands, *Ugeskr Laeger, 153(12),* 833-835.

[31] Kuusi, M., Hasseltvedt, V., Aavitsland, P. (1999). Surveillance Report: Botulism in Norway. *Eurosurveillance, Jan;4(1):*11-12.

[32] Schjonsby, H. P. (2002). Botulisme I Osterdalen I 1831. *Medisinsk Historie, 122*, 2860-2862.

[33] Jensen, T., Jacobsen, D., van der Lippe, E., Yndestad, M. (1998). Botulism after intake of half fermented Fish, *Tidsskr Nor Laegeforen, 118(28),* 4366-4367.

[34] Kazdobina, I.S., Terekhova, E.B., Podunova, L.G., Vertiev, Y.V. (1995). Botulism in the Russian Federation: 1988 -1922, *Zhurnal Mikrobiologii, Epidemiologii, Immunobiologii, 6*, 98-99.

[35] Mazurin, N,D., Gelman, E.I., Perminov, V.G., Ulitskil, L.A., Kishko, Z.B. (1967). On Cases of type E Botulism on Kamchatka, *Zhurnal Mikrobiologli, Epidemiologii, Immunobiologii, 44(12),* 122-125.

[36] Mazurin, N,D., & Merzliakov, A.P (1967). On Cases of type E Botulism on Sakhalin, *Zhurnal Mikrobiologli, Epidemiologii, Immunobiologii, 44(3),* 123-125.

[37] Ball, A. P., Hopkinson, R. B., Farrell, I. D., Hutchinson, J. G. P., Paul, R. Watson, R. D., S., et al. (1979). Human Botulism Caused by Clostridium Botulinum Type E: The Birmingham Outbreak, *Quarterly Journal of Medicine, 191*, 473-491.

[38] Fagan, R.P., McLaughlin, J. B., & Middaugh, J.P. (2009). Persistence of Botulinum Toxin in Patients' Serum: Alaska, 1959-2007. *Journal of Infectious Diseases 199*, 1029-1031.

[39] Hayes, A. H. (1983). The Food and Drug Administration's Role in the Canned Salmon Recalls of 1982. *Public Health Reports, 98*, 412-415.

[40] Korkeala, H., Stengel, G., Hyytia, E., Vogelsang, B., Bohl, A., Wihlman, H., et al. (1998). Type E botulism associated with vacuum-packaged hot-smoked whitefish, *Int J Food Microbiology 18(43),* 1-5.

[41] Hyytia, E., Hielm, S., Bjorkroth, J., & Korkeala, H. (1999). Biodiversity of *Clostridium botulinum* Type E Strains Isolated from Fish and Fishery Products. *Applied and Environmental Microbiology, 65(5)*, 2057-2064.

[42] Lindstrom, M. Vuorela, M. Hinderink, K., Korkeala, H. Dahlsten, E., Raahenmaa K, et al. (2006). Botulism associated with vacuum-packed smoked whitefish in Finland. *Eurosurveillance, 29*. Jul 20;11(7).

[43] King, L.A., Niskanen, T., Junnikkala, M., MoiLanen,E., Lindstrom, M., Korkeala, H, et al. (2009). Botulism and Hot-smoked Whitefish: A Family Cluster of Type E Botulism in France, September 2009. *Eurosurveillance,14*, 45.

ISBN: 978-1-63483-384-4

Bibliography

A practical guide to botulinum toxin procedures LCCN: 2011015537 Small, Rebecca. A practical guide to botulinum toxin procedures / Rebecca Small; associate editor, Dalano Hoang. Published/Created: Philadelphia: Wolters Kluwer/Lippincott Williams & Wilkins Health, c2012. Description: xi, 155 p.: col ill.; 26 cm. ISBN: 9781609131470 (alk. paper) 1609131479 (alk. paper) LC classification: RL120.B66 S63 2012 Related names: Hoang, Dalano. Contents: Frown lines -- Horizontal forehead lines -- Crow's feet -- Lower eyelid wrinkles -- Eyebrow lift -- Bunny lines -- Lip lines -- Gummy smile -- Marionette lines -- Chin -- Neck bands -- Axillary hyperhidrosis. Subjects: Botulinum toxin--Therapeutic use. Injections, Intradermal. Botulinum Toxins--therapeutic use--Handbooks. Cosmetic Techniques--Handbooks. Injections, Intradermal--methods--Handbooks. Notes: Includes bibliographical references (p. 147-150) and index. Dewey class no.615/.778.

Anal fissure: symptoms, diagnosis and treatment LCCN: 2011009052 Anal fissure: symptoms, diagnosis and treatment / editors, Pierpaolo Sileri and Achille Lucio Gaspari. Published/Created: Hauppauge, N.Y.: Nova Science Publishers, c2012. Description: x, 130 p.: ill.; 23 cm. ISBN: 9781612097169 (softcover: alk. paper) LC classification: RC866 .A53 2012 Related names: Sileri, Pierpaolo. Gaspari, Achille. Contents: Anal canal: anatomy, physiopathology and diagnosis / Michele Grande -- Chemical sphincterotomy /

Giovanni Milito, Federica Cadeddu -- Botulinum toxin and anal fissure / Oliver Jones -- Current surgical management / Herand Abcarian and Jason W. Allen -- Postoperative complications after treatment for chronic anal fissure / Federica Cadeddu -- Anal fissure: treatment options in particular cases / Stefano D'Ugo ... [et al.] -- Conservative and surgical treatment of chronic anal fissure: longer-term results from our prospective database / Pierpaolo Sileri ... [et al.]. Subjects: Anus--Diseases. Anus--Diseases--Treatment. Fissure in Ano--therapy. Fissure in Ano--diagnosis. Notes: Includes bibliographical references and index. Series: Public health in the 21st century Dewey class no.: 616.3/5

Botulinum neurotoxins LCCN: 2012952294 Botulinum neurotoxins / Andreas Rummel, Thomas Binz, editors. Published/Created: Heidelberg; New York: Springer, c2013. Description: viii, 321 p.: ill. (some col.); 24 cm. ISBN: 9783642335693 (alk. paper) 3642335691 (alk. paper) 9783642335709 (ebk.) LC classification: QP632.B66 B68 2013 RC350.C54 Related names: Rummel, Andreas. Binz, Thomas. Summary: The extremely potent substance botulinum neurotoxin (BoNT) has attracted much interest in diverse fields. Originally identified as cause for the rare but deadly disease botulism, military and terrorist intended to misuse this sophisticated molecule as biological weapon. This caused its classification as select agent category A by the Centers for Diseases Control and Prevention and the listing in the Biological and Toxin Weapons Convention. Later, the civilian use of BoNT as long acting peripheral muscle relaxant has turned this molecule into an indispensable pharmaceutical world wide with annual revenues >$1.5 billion-- Source other than Library of Congress. Contents: Genetic diversity within Clostridium botulinum serotypes, botulinum neurotoxin gene clusters and toxin subtypes / Karen K. Hill and Theresa J. Smith -- Assembly and function of the botulinum neurotoxin progenitor complex / Shenyan Gu and Rongsheng Jin -- Uptake of botulinum neurotoxin in the intestine / Yukako Fujinage, Yo Sugawara and Takuhiro Matsumura -- Double receptor anchorage of botulinum neurotoxins accounts for their exquisite neurospecificity /

Andreas Rummel -- The elusive compass of clostridial neurotoxins: Deciding when and where to go? / Kinga Bercsenyi, Francesco Giribaldi and Giampietro Schiavo -- Synchronized chaperone function of botulinum neurotoxin domains mediates light chain translocation into neurons / Audrey Fischer -- Clostridial neurotoxin light chains: Devices for SNARE cleavage mediated blockade of neurotransmission / Thomas Binz -- Synaptic vesicle proteins: Targets and routes for botulinum neurotoxins / Gudrun Ahnert-Hilger, Agnieszka Münster-Wandowski and Markus Höltje -- Persistence of botulinum neurotoxin inactivation of nerve function / Charles B. Shoemaker and George A. Oyler -- Structure-based drug discovery for botulinum neurotoxins / Subramanyam Swaminathan -- Complexity of botulinum neurotoxins: Challenges for detection technology / Martin B. Dorner ... [et al.] -- Progress in cell based assays for botulinum neurotoxin detection / Sabine Pellett -- Transforming the domain structure of botulinum neurotoxins into novel therapeutics / John Chaddock -- Botulinum toxin: Application, safety, and limitations / Hans Bigalke. Subjects: Botulinum toxin. Botulinum toxin--Therapeutic use. Botulinum Toxins, Type A--therapeutic use. Botulinum Toxins, Type A--pharmacology. Neuromuscular Agents--pharmacology. Neuromuscular Agents--therapeutic use. Botulinum toxin -- Therapeutic use. Botulinum Toxins -- therapeutic use. Toxines botuliniques. Toxines botuliniques--Emploi en thérapeutique. Subject keywords: Clostridium Notes: Includes bibliographical references and index. Series: Current topics in microbiology and immunology, 0070-217X; v.364 Current topics in microbiology and immunology; 364. 0070-217X Dewey class no.: 615.9/5 615.95

Botulinum neurotoxins LCCN: 2012952294 Botulinum neurotoxins / Andreas Rummel, Thomas Binz, editors. Published/Created: Heidelberg; New York: Springer, c2013. Description: viii, 321 p.: ill. (some col.); 24 cm. ISBN: 9783642335693 (alk. paper) 3642335691 (alk. paper) 9783642335709 (ebk.) LC classification: QP632.B66 B68 2013 RC350.C54 Related names: Rummel, Andreas. Binz,

Thomas. Summary: The extremely potent substance botulinum neurotoxin (BoNT) has attracted much interest in diverse fields. Originally identified as cause for the rare but deadly disease botulism, military and terrorist intended to misuse this sophisticated molecule as biological weapon. This caused its classification as select agent category A by the Centers for Diseases Control and Prevention and the listing in the Biological and Toxin Weapons Convention. Later, the civilian use of BoNT as long acting peripheral muscle relaxant has turned this molecule into an indispensable pharmaceutical world wide with annual revenues >$1.5 billion-- Source other than Library of Congress. Contents: Genetic diversity within Clostridium botulinum serotypes, botulinum neurotoxin gene clusters and toxin subtypes / Karen K. Hill and Theresa J. Smith -- Assembly and function of the botulinum neurotoxin progenitor complex / Shenyan Gu and Rongsheng Jin -- Uptake of botulinum neurotoxin in the intestine / Yukako Fujinage, Yo Sugawara and Takuhiro Matsumura -- Double receptor anchorage of botulinum neurotoxins accounts for their exquisite neurospecificity / Andreas Rummel -- The elusive compass of clostridial neurotoxins: Deciding when and where to go? / Kinga Bercsenyi, Francesco Giribaldi and Giampietro Schiavo -- Synchronized chaperone function of botulinum neurotoxin domains mediates light chain translocation into neurons / Audrey Fischer -- Clostridial neurotoxin light chains: Devices for SNARE cleavage mediated blockade of neurotransmission / Thomas Binz -- Synaptic vesicle proteins: Targets and routes for botulinum neurotoxins / Gudrun Ahnert-Hilger, Agnieszka Münster-Wandowski and Markus Höltje -- Persistence of botulinum neurotoxin inactivation of nerve function / Charles B. Shoemaker and George A. Oyler -- Structure-based drug discovery for botulinum neurotoxins / Subramanyam Swaminathan -- Complexity of botulinum neurotoxins: Challenges for detection technology / Martin B. Dorner ... [et al.] -- Progress in cell based assays for botulinum neurotoxin detection / Sabine Pellett -- Transforming the domain structure of botulinum neurotoxins into novel therapeutics / John Chaddock -- Botulinum toxin: Application, safety, and limitations / Hans Bigalke. Subjects: Botulinum toxin. Botulinum toxin--Therapeutic use. Botulinum Toxins, Type A--therapeutic use. Botulinum Toxins, Type A--pharmacology. Neuromuscular Agents--pharmacology. Neuromuscular Agents--therapeutic use. Botulinum toxin -- Therapeutic use. Botulinum Toxins -- therapeutic use. Toxines botuliniques. Toxines botuliniques--Emploi en thérapeutique. Subject keywords: Clostridium Notes: Includes bibliographical references and index. Series: Current topics in microbiology and immunology, 0070-217X; v.364 Current topics in microbiology and immunology; 364. 0070-217X Dewey class no.: 615.9/5 615.95

Botulinum toxin: uses, mechanisms of action and complications LCCN: 2012939702 Botulinum toxin: uses, mechanisms of action and complications / [edited by] Fausto E. Marino, Sebastiano De Luca. Published/Created: Hauppauge, NY: Nova Science Publishers, Inc., 2012. Description: p. cm. ISBN: 9781622571857 (hardcover)

Botulinum toxin in dermatology: a clinical overview LCCN: 2014958715 Botulinum toxin in dermatology: a clinical overview / [edited by] Anna Campanati, Annamaria Offidani. Published/Produced: Hauppauge, NY: Nova Science Publishers, Inc., 2015. Description: pages cm ISBN: 9781634638128 (softcover)

Botulinum toxin LCCN: 2012540520 Botulinum toxin / edited by Alastair Carruthers, Jean Carruthers. Edition: 3rd ed. Published/Created: London: Saunders Elsevier, 2013. Description: xiv, 183 p.: ill.; 27 cm. ISBN: 9781455727810 1455727814 9781455737765 (Ebook) 1455737763 (Ebook) LC classification: QP632.B66 B69 2013 Related names: Carruthers, Alastair. Carruthers, Jean. Subjects: Botulinum toxin. Botulinum Toxins, Type A--therapeutic use. Cosmetic Techniques. Face. Neck. Notes: Includes bibliographical references and index. Series: Procedures in cosmetic dermatology Procedures in cosmetic dermatology.

Clostridium botulinum: a spore forming organism and a challenge to food safety LCCN: 2011024362 Clostridium botulinum: a spore forming organism and a challenge to food safety / Christine Rasetti-Escargueil and Susanne Surman-Lee, editors. Published/Created: New York: Nova Science Publishers, c2012. Description: x, 278 p.: ill.; 24 cm. ISBN: 9781614705758 (hardcover) 1614705755 (hardcover) LC classification: QR201.B7 C55 2012 Related names: Rasetti-Escargueil, Christine. Surman-Lee, Susanne. Contents: Clostridium botulinum: history, strains, and neurotoxin diversity / Michel Popoff and Mazuet Christelle -- The molecular and structural biology of Clostridium botulinum neurotoxins reveals insights into the sophisticated mechanism of neurotoxicity / Andreas Rummel -- History of botulism: botulism around the world in the 20th century / Zane Horowitz -- Infant botulism / Lucia Fenicia, Fabrizio Anniballi -- Passage of botulinum toxins through the intestinal barrier / Yukako Fujinaga -- Botulism symptoms, incubation period, complications, diagnosis, and management / Itzhak Brook -- Botulism hazards from native foods in the Arctic regions / B. Zane Horowitz -- Detecting botulinum in food: effective and sensitive detection of Clostridium botulinum toxin in foods / Uma Basavanna, Guy E. Skinner, and Shashi K. Sharma -- Integrated approach used by government agencies and industry to protect the consumer: food safety legislation / Angela Iriajen, C. Rasetti-Escargueil -- Control in primary food production: meat, fish, and vegetables. Control in processed foods: meat products, fish products, vegetable products, and dairy products. Control in REPFEDS / Angela Iriajen -- Safe process design and food hygiene guidelines / Flavio L. Schmidt -- Predictive modelling: predicting exposure of consumers to Clostridium botulinum neurotoxin in processed food / Pradeep Malakar. Subjects: Botulism. Clostridium botulinum. Food--Microbiology. Food--Safety measures. Botulism--etiology. Botulinum Toxins--adverse effects. Botulism--prevention & control. Clostridium botulinum--pathogenicity. Food Handling--standards. Food Safety--methods. Notes: Includes bibliographical references and index. Series: Advances in food safety and food microbiology Advances in food safety and food microbiology. Dewey class no.: 615.9/5293

Cosmetic and clinical applications of botox and dermal fillers LCCN: 2015002457 Lipham, William J., 1964-, author. Cosmetic and clinical applications of botox and dermal fillers / William J. Lipham, Jill S. Melicher. Edition: Third edition. Published/Produced: Thorofare, NJ: SLACK Incorporated, 2015. Description: xvi, 142 pages; 27 cm ISBN: 9781617110856 (hardback) LC classification: RL120.B66 L55 2015 Related names: Melicher, Jill S., editor. Summary: "This book is for medical personnel interested in the use of BOTOX and dermal filler agents for a wide variety of functional and minimally invasive facial rejuvenation procedures"-- Provided by publisher. Contents: A brief history of the clinical applications of botulinum toxin / William J. Lipham -- What is botulinum toxin and how does it work? / William J. Lipham and Jill S. Melicher -- Pertinent facial muscle anatomy / William J. Lipham -- Getting started: commercially available products, basic equipment and supplies, reconstitution and dilution recommendations, and clinical implementation / William J. Lipham and Jill S. Melicher -- Treatment of blepharospasm, Meige syndrome, and hemifacial spasm / William J. Lipham -- Botulinum toxin as a treatment for functional disorders / Michael S. McCracken, David B. Granet, and Don O. Kikkawa -- Neuro-Ophthalmic uses for botulinum toxin / Patrick K. Johnson, David B. Granet, and William J. Lipham -- Cosmetic applications of botulinum toxin / William J. Lipham and Jill S. Melicher -- Periorbital rejuvenation using cosmetic filler agents and fat Injection / Greg S. Gayre, David R. Jordan, and William J. Lipham -- Marketing botulinum toxin and dermal filler agents to build your practice / William J. Lipham and Jill S. Melicher. Subjects: Botulinum Toxins, Type A--therapeutic use. Cosmetic Techniques. Facial Muscles--drug effects. Notes: Includes bibliographical references and index. Dewey class no.: 615.7/78

Hankey's clinical neurology LCCN: 2014395481 Clinical neurology (Hankey) Hankey's clinical neurology / editors, Philip B. Gorelick, MD, MPH, FACP, FAHA, FAAN, FANA, Medical Director, Mercy Health Hauenstein Neuroscience Center at Saint Mary's, Professor, Translational Science &

Molecular Medicine, Michigan State University College of Human Medicine, Grand Rapids, Michigan, USA, Fernando D. Testai, MD, PhD, FAHA, Assistant Professor in Neurology, University of Illinois College Medicine at Chicago, Chicago, Illinois, USA, Graeme J. Hankey, MBBS, MD, FRACP, FRCP, FRCPE, Winthrop Professor of Neurology, School of Medicine and Pharmacology, The University of Western Australia, Consultant Neurologist, Department of Neurology, Sir Charles Gairdner Hospital, Perth, Australia, Joanna M. Wardlaw, MBChB, MRCP, DMRD, FRCR, MD, FRCP, FMedSc, Professor of Applied Neuroimaging, Division of Clinical Neurosciences, University of Edinburgh, Western General Hospital, Edinburgh, UK. Edition: Second edition. Published/Created: Boca Raton: CRC Press/Taylor & Francis Group, [2014] Description: 975 pages: illustrations (chiefly color); 27 cm ISBN: 9781840761931 (hardback: acid-free paper) 1840761938 (hardback: acid-free paper) LC classification: RC346 .H2356 2014 Portion of title: Clinical neurology Related names: Gorelick, Philip B. Testai, Fernando D. Hankey, Graeme J. Wardlaw, Joanna M. Contents: Machine generated contents note: ch. 1 Neurologic diagnosis / Robert Edis -- Introduction -- The diagnostic process in neurology -- Neurologic examination -- Lumbar puncture and CSF examination / John Dunne -- Neurophysiologic examination / William McAuliffe -- Imaging the brain and spine -- ch. 2 Disorders of consciousness / Venkatesh Aiyagari -- Impaired consciousness -- Brain death -- Persistent/permanent vegetative state -- Minimally conscious state -- Locked-in syndrome -- Syncope -- Hypoxic--ischemic encephalopathy -- Central pontine myelinolysis -- ch. 3 Epilepsy / Andres M. Kanner -- Definition -- Epidemiology -- Pathophysiology -- Classification -- Clinical features -- Differential diagnosis -- Investigation and diagnosis -- Treatment -- ch. 4 Headache / Peter J. Goadsby -- Headache -- Migraine -- Tension-type headache -- Cluster headache -- ch. 5 Vertigo / Jorge Kattah -- Introduction -- Specific syndromes -- ch. 6 Hyperkinetic movement disorders / Philip Thompson -- Contents note continued: Introduction -- Dystonia -- Chorea -- Tremor --

Myoclonus -- Tics -- Stereotypies -- Dyskinesias -- Drug-induced movement disorders -- Psychogenic movement disorders -- ch. 7 Developmental diseases of the nervous system / James H. Tonsgard -- Introduction -- Embryonic development of the nervous system -- Developmental malformations of the nervous system -- Defects in neural tube formation -- Defects in hindbrain development -- Defects in forebrain and cerebral development -- Neurocutaneous disorders -- Neurofibromatosis Type 1 -- Neurofibromatosis Type 2 -- Tuberous sclerosis -- Sturge--Weber syndrome -- Hereditary hemorrhagic telangiectasia (Osler--Rendu--Weber syndrome) -- Linear nevus sebaceous syndrome -- Cowden's syndrome and Lhermitte--Duclos disease -- von Hippel--Lindau disease -- Incontinentia pigmenti -- Hypomelanosis of Ito -- ch. 8 Hereditary and metabolic diseases of the central nervous system in adults / Alma R. Bicknese -- Introduction -- Contents note continued: Metabolic and degenerative diseases in adults -- Huntington's disease -- Cerebral autosomal dominant arteriopathy with subcortical infarcts and leukoencephalopathy -- Fragile X-associated tremor/ataxia syndrome -- X-linked adrenoleukodystrophy -- Pantothenate kinase-associated neurodegeneration -- Inherited diseases with prominent visceral and neurologic findings -- Wilson's disease -- Acute intermittent porphyria -- Disorders of amino acid metabolism -- Homocystinuria -- Inclusion body disorders -- Lafora body disease -- Adult neuronal ceroid lipofuscinoses -- Late-onset lysosomal storage diseases -- Late-onset GM2 gangliosidosis -- Late-onset metachromatic leukodystrophy -- Fabry's disease -- Late-onset Krabbe disease -- Niemann--Pick Type C -- Mitochondrial disorders -- Diseases of mitochondrial DNA -- ch. 9 Trauma of the brain and spinal cord / Prasad S.S.V. Vannemreddy -- Introduction -- Head injury -- Concussion -- Spinal cord injury -- Contents note continued: ch. 10 Stroke and transient ischemic attacks of the brain and eye / Graeme J. Hankey -- Introduction -- Epidemiology -- Pathology and etiology -- Risk factors -- Clinical assessment -- Investigations -- Diagnosis -- Prognosis -- Treatment -- ch. 11

Infections of the central nervous system / James L. Cook -- Acute bacterial meningitis -- Brain abscess -- Neurosyphilis -- Lyme disease -- Tuberculosis (TB) -- Botulism -- Tetanus -- Aseptic meningitis -- Viral encephalitis -- Rabies -- Poliomyelitis -- Progressive multifocal leukoencephalopathy (PML) -- Cryptococcosis -- Coccidioidomycosis -- Toxoplasmosis -- Neurocysticercosis -- Eosinophilic meningitis -- Creutzfeldt--Jakob disease (CJD) -- ch. 12 Inflammatory disorders of the nervous system / Neil Scolding -- Acute disseminated encephalomyelitis (post-infectious encephalomyelitis) -- Multiple sclerosis (MS) -- Neurosarcoidosis -- Cavernous sinus syndrome -- Contents note continued: ch. 13 Tumors of the nervous system / Robert P. Dinapoli -- Neoplasia -- Gliomas -- Meningioma -- Craniopharyngioma -- Pituitary tumors -- Vestibular schwannoma (acoustic neuroma) -- Primary central nervous system lymphoma -- Germ cell tumors of the CNS -- von Hippel--Lindau disease -- Metastases to the CNS -- Paraneoplastic neurologic disease -- ch. 14 Degenerative diseases of the nervous system / James A. Mastrianni -- Dementia -- Alzheimer's disease (AD) -- Frontotemporal dementia (FTD) -- Dementia with Lewy bodies (DLB) -- Vascular dementia -- Prion diseases -- Normal pressure hydrocephalus / Kathleen M. Shannon -- Parkinson's disease and parkinsonian disorders -- Introduction -- Primary (idiopathic) parkinsonism: Parkinson's disease -- Multisystem degenerations (Parkinsonism plus' or atypical parkinsonism) -- Heredodegenerative and secondary parkinsonism / Peter Todd -- Hereditary ataxias -- Introduction -- Congenital ataxias -- Contents note continued: Autosomal dominant cerebellar ataxias -- Autosomal recessive cerebellar ataxias -- X-linked causes of ataxia -- ch. 15 Acquired metabolic diseases of the nervous system / Fernando D. Testai -- Thiamine deficiency: Wernick--Korsakoff syndrome -- Vitamin B12 deficiency -- Vitamin E deficiency -- Niacin (nicotinic acid) deficiency -- Marchiafava--Bignami disease -- Hepatic encephalopathy -- Uremic encephalopathy -- Posterior reversible encephalopathy syndrome -- ch. 16 Disorders of circulation of the cerebrospinal fluid / Edward A. Michals -- Introduction -- Aqueductal stenosis with hydrocephalus -- Communicating hydrocepahalus -- Normal pressure hydrocephalus -- Chiari malformation -- Syringomyelia (syringohydromyelia) -- Idiopathic intracranial hypertension (pseudotumor cerebri) -- Intracranial hypotension syndrome -- ch. 17 Cranial neuropathies I, V, and VII--XII / Helene Rubeiz -- Olfactory nerve neuropathy (cranial nerve I) -- Contents note continued: Trigeminal nerve neuropathy (cranial nerve V) -- Selected conditions affecting the trigeminal nerve -- Facial nerve neuropathy (cranial nerve VII) -- Selected conditions affecting the facial nerve -- Vestibulo-cochlear nerve neuropathy (cranial nerve VIII) -- Glossopharyngeal nerve neuropathy (cranial nerve IX) -- Selected conditions affecting the glossopharyngeal nerve -- Vagus nerve neuropathy (cranial nerve X) -- Spinal accessory nerve neuropathy (cranial nerve XI) -- Hypoglossal nerve neuropathy (cranial nerve XII) -- ch. 18 Cranial neuropathies II, III, IV, and VI / Molly E. Gilbert -- Optic nerve neuropathy (cranial nerve II) -- Cranial nerve III, IV, and VI palsies -- ch. 19 Spinal cord disease / Octavia Kincaid -- Introduction to myelopathy -- Extramedullar spinal cord lesions (extrinsic myelopathy) -- Intramedullary spinal cord lesions (intrinsic myelopathy) -- Inflammatory myelopathy (e.g., myelitis) -- Infectious myelopathy -- Contents note continued: Metabolic and toxic myelopathies -- Vascular myelopathies -- Structural myelopathies -- Hereditary myelopathies -- Spinal cord tumors -- Myelopathy associated with motor neuron disease -- ch. 20 Autonomic nervous system disorders / Judy Spies -- Autonomic neuropathy -- ch. 21 Diseases of the peripheral nerve and mononeuropathies / Andrea Swenson -- Peripheral neuropathy -- Diabetic neuropathy -- Toxic neuropathy -- Nutrition-related neuropathy -- Neuropathy in systemic disease -- Guillain--Barre syndrome (GBS)/Acute inflammatory demyelinating polyradiculoneuropathy (AIDP) -- Chronic acquired demyelinating polyneuropathy -- Vasculitic neuropathy -- Immune-mediated brachial plexus neuropathy (IBPN) -- Infectious neuropathy -- Hereditary motor and sensory neuropathy (Charcot--Marie--

Tooth disease) -- Syndromic hereditary peripheral neuropathies -- Mononeuropathies -- Upper extremity neuropathy -- Lower extremity neuropathy -- Contents note continued: ch. 22 Neuromuscular junction disorders / Julie Rowin -- Myasthenia gravis -- Congenital myasthenic syndromes -- Lambert--Eaton myasthenic syndrome -- Botulism -- ch. 23 Muscle disorders / Betty Soliven -- Introduction -- Myopathy -- Inflammatory myopathy -- Critical illness myopathy -- Endocrine and metabolic myopathies -- Muscular dystrophies -- Muscle channelopathies (disorders of membrane excitability) -- ch. 24 Sleep disorders / Michael Kohrman -- Introduction -- Normal sleep -- Commonly performed sleep tests -- Insomnias -- Hypersomnias of central origin -- Sleep-related movement disorders -- Sleep-related breathing disorders -- Circadian rhythm sleep disorders -- Parasomnias -- Conclusion. Subjects: Neurology. Nervous system--Diseases. Notes: Includes bibliographical references and index. Dewey class no.: •616.8

Illustrated guide to aesthetic botulinum toxic injections: basics, indications, uses LCCN: 2014378846 Kane, Michael A. C., author. Illustrated guide to aesthetic botulinum toxic injections: basics, indications, uses / Michael Kane, Gerhard Sattler; with 274 illustrations. Published/Produced: London: Quintessence, 2013. Description: 160 pages: illustrations; 24 cm. Links: http://d-nb.info/1043758445/04 Inhaltsverzeichnis ISBN: 9781850972501 (hbk.) 1850972508 (hbk.) Related names: Sattler, G. (Gerhard), 1955- author. Subjects: Surgery, Plastic. Botulinum toxin. Series: Aesthetic methods for skin rejuvenation series

Manual of botulinum toxin therapy LCCN: 2013014807 Manual of botulinum toxin therapy / [edited by] Daniel Truong ... [et al.]. Edition: 2nd ed. Published/Created: Cambridge, UK; New York: Cambridge University Press, 2013. Description: xiii, 305 p.: ill.; 26 cm. ISBN: 9781107025356 (hardback) LC classification: RL120.B66 M36 2013 Related names: Truong, Daniel, M.D. Summary: "This book tries to answer many of the questions posed above with the contributions of a team of international experts. As in the first edition, the emphasis in this book is on technique, so it is richly endowed with illustrations concerning accurate access techniques to help physicians become facile and fully competent"--Provided by publisher. Subjects: Botulinum Toxins--therapeutic use. Neuromuscular Agents--therapeutic use. Botulinum Toxins--pharmacology. Movement Disorders--drug therapy. Neuromuscular Diseases--drug therapy. Notes: Includes bibliographical references and index. Dewey class no.: 615/.778

Non-invasive cosmetic procedures: Thomas procedures in facial plastic surgery LCCN: 2011033035 Non-invasive cosmetic procedures: Thomas procedures in facial plastic surgery / [edited by] R. James Koch. Published/Created: Shelton, CT: People's Medical Pub. House, 2012. Description: ix, 102 p.: ill. (some col.); 26 cm. ISBN: 9781607951506 1607951509 LC classification: RD119.5.F33 N66 2012 Related names: Koch, R. James. Contents: Soft tissue fillers / Jeffrey D. Pollard, Thomas H. Moulthrop, Calvin M. Johnson Jr. -- Botulinum toxin / Jeffrey D. Pollard, Thomas H. Moulthrop, Calvin M. Johnson Jr. -- Laser skin resurfacing / Vishal Banthia, Basil M. Hantash, James Koch -- Non-ablative lasers and lights / Vishal Banthia, Basil M. Hantash, James Koch -- Laser skin tightening / Basil M. Hantash, R. James Koch, Brian Kim -- Radiofrequency tissue tightening / R. James Koch, Brian Kim -- Microdermabrasion / Matthew Hanasono, R. James Koch -- Chemical peels / Vishal Banthia, Basil M. Hantash, R. James Koch -- Cosmeceuticals / Mary Lynn Moran. Subjects: Face--Surgery. Surgery, Plastic. Face--surgery. Cosmetic Techniques. Reconstructive Surgical Procedures--methods. Surgical Procedures, Minimally Invasive--methods. Notes: Includes bibliographical references and index. Series: Thomas procedures in facial plastic surgery Dewey class no.: 617.5/2059

Orofacial pain: a guide to medications and management LCCN: 2011036432 Clark, Glenn T. Orofacial pain: a guide to medications and management / editors: Glenn T. Clark, Raymond A. Dionne. Published/Created: Chichester,

West Sussex, UK; Ames, Iowa: Wiley-Blackwell, 2012. Description: vii, 400 p.: ill. (some col.); 28 cm. ISBN: 9780813815596 (pbk.: alk. paper) 0813815592 (pbk.: alk. paper) LC classification: RK322 .C58 2012 Related names: Dionne, Raymond. Summary: "Pain is a preoccupation in dentistry, but the dentist's role has expanded beyond the treatment of dental pain to being one of the most involved in the treatment of orofacial pain. Orofacial Pain: A Guide to Medications and Management guides readers through the rational use of medications for the treatment of chronic orofacial pain, including oral, injectable and topical medications. It also provides relevant information about treatment choices for managing neuropathic and musculoskeletal pain, headache and uncommon orofacial pain disorders"--Provided by publisher. Contents: The top 30 chronic painful diseases, disorders, and dysfunctions that occur in the orofacial region / Glenn T. Clark -- Top 60 most important medications used in an OFP treatment center / Glenn T. Clark -- Non-opioid analgesics, salicylates, NSAIDs, and corticosteroids for chronic pain / Raymond A. Dionne, Glenn T. Clark -- Opioids for chronic orofacial pain with a focus on non-malignant chronic pain / Glenn T. Clark, Steven H. Richeimer -- Nocebo responsive patients and topical pain control agents used for orofacial and mucosal pain / Glenn T. Clark -- Anti-convulsants agents used for neuropathic pain including trigeminal neuralgia / Glenn T. Clark, Antonia Teruel -- Skeletal muscle relaxants and anti-spasticity drugs for orofacial pain disorders / Glenn Clark, Soma Sahai-Srivastava -- Psychopharmacologic agents (antidepressants, antipsychotics, anxiolytics, and psychostimulants) used in chronic pain / Glenn T. Clark ... [et al.] -- Anti-bacterial agents as analgesics in chronic pain / Satish Kumar, Glenn T. Clark, Raymond A. Dionne -- Using oral medications, infusions, and injections for differential diagnosis of orofacial pain / Saravanan Ram, Satish Kumar, Glenn T. Clark -- Interventional therapy and injected agents for orofacial pain and spasm (including botulinum toxin) / Glenn T. Clark, Alan Stiles -- Treatment for oral mucositis and non-infectious, non-neoplastic oral ulcerations / Satish Kumar, Antonia Teruel, Glenn T. Clark -

- Management of orofacial pain and other co-morbidities in oropharyngeal and nasopharyngeal cancer patients / Saravanan Ram, Glenn T. Clark -- Burning mouth syndrome: an update on diagnosis and treatment methods / Piedad Suarez Durall, Glenn T. Clark -- Headaches with a focus on chronic daily HA medications / Soma Sahai-Srivastava, Glenn Clark -- Differential diagnosis and management of masticatory myogenous pain and dysfunction / Glenn T. Clark -- Diagnosing and managing chronic trigeminal neuropathy / Glenn T. Clark -- Temporomandibular joint arthritis: implications, diagnosis, and management / Antonia Teruel, Jack S. Broussard Jr., Glenn T. Clark -- Five oral motor disorders: habitual tooth clenching and other involuntary oral motor disorders / Glenn T. Clark, Saravanan Ram -- Diagnosis and treatment of TMJ internal derangements / Glenn T. Clark. Subjects: Orofacial pain--Treatment. Facial pain--Treatment. Facial Pain--drug therapy. Facial Pain--prevention & control. Analgesics--therapeutic use. Chronic Disease. Facial Neuralgia. Notes: Includes bibliographical references and index. Dewey class no.: 615.1/9

Practical psychodermatology LCCN: 2013042712 Practical psychodermatology / [edited by] Anthony Bewley, Ruth E. Taylor, Jason S. Reichenberg, Michelle Magid; foreword by Dr John Koo, Dr Christopher Brigett, and Dr Richard Staughton. Published/Produced: Chichester, West Sussex, UK: John Wiley and Sons, Inc., 2014. Description: p.; cm. ISBN: 9781118560686 (cloth) LC classification: RL96 Related names: Bewley, Anthony, editor of compilation. Taylor, Ruth E., editor of compilation. Reichenberg, Jason S., editor of compilation. Magid, Michelle, editor of compilation. Contents: Introduction to psychodermatology / Anthony Bewley, Ruth Taylor, Jason S. Reichenberg, and Michelle Magid -- Psychodermatology: history and examination / Anthony Bewley, Ruth Taylor, Jason S. Reichenberg, and Michelle Magid -- Psychopharmacology in psychodermatology / Michelle Magid, Sussann Kotara, and Maureen Burrows -- Psychological assessment and interventions for people with skin disease / Reena B. Shahÿ -- Risk analysis, management, and the Mental Health Act / Simon Kirwin -- Psychological impact of hair loss / Paul Farrant and Sue McHale -- Psoriasis and psychodermatology / Chris Bundy, Lis Cordingley, and Chris Griffiths -- Adherence in the treatment of chronic skin diseases / Laura F. Sandoval, Christine S. Ahn, and Steven R. Feldman -- Living well with a skin condition: what it takes / Henrietta Spalding, Wendy Eastwood, Krysia Saul, and Susan Bradbrooke -- Chronic skin disease and anxiety, depression, and other affective disorders / Steve Reid and Wojcik Wojtek -- Self-help for management of psychological distress associated with skin conditions / Andrew R. Thompson -- Delusional infestation / Peter Lepping, Roland Freudenmann, and Markus Huber -- Body dysmorphic disorder / Emma Baldock and David Veale -- Dysesthetic syndromes / Sara A. Hylwa, Mark D.P. Davis, and Mark R. Pittelkow -- Chronic idiopathic mucocutaneous pain syndromes: vulvodynia, penodynia and scrotodynia / Peter J. Lynch and Libby Edwards -- Burning mouth syndrome / Alison Bruce, Rochelle Torgerson, and Tania Gonzalez Santiago -- Medically unexplained symptoms (MUS) & health anxieties: somatic symptom and related disorders / Angharad Ruttley, Audrey Ng, and Anna Burnside -- Nodular prurigo / Wei Sheng Tan, Hong Liang Tey, and Mark B.Y. Tang -- Pickers, pokers, and pullers: obsessive-compulsive related disorders in dermatology / Jonathan S. Abramowitz and Ryan J. Jacoby -- Habit reversal therapy: a behavioral approach to atopic eczema, and other skin conditions / Christopher Bridgett -- Child and adolescent psychodermatology / Birgit Westphal and Osman Malik -- Nursing interventions in psychodermatology / Fiona Cowdell and Steven Ersser -- Psychological reactions to skin cancer / Andrew Affleck and Lesley Howells -- Factitious skin disorder (dermatitis artefacta) / Leslie Millard -- Botulinum toxin treatment in depression / M. Axel Wollmer, Michelle Magid and Tillmann Kruger -- The morgellons debate / Michelle Magid and Jason S. Reichenberg -- Substance misuse and the dermatology patient / Alexander Verner. Subjects: Skin Diseases--psychology. Mental Disorders--etiology. Mental Disorders--therapy. Psychophysiologic Disorders--therapy. Skin Diseases--complications. Skin Manifestations. Notes: Includes bibliographical references and index. Additional formats: Online version: Practical psychodermatology Chichester, West Sussex, UK: John Wiley and Sons, Inc., 2014 9781118560679 (DLC) 2013043949 Dewey class no.: 616.5/0651

Principles of deglutition: a multidisciplinary text for swallowing and its disorders LCCN: 2012943384 Principles of deglutition: a multidisciplinary text for swallowing and its disorders / Reza Shaker ... [et al.], editors. Published/Created: New York: Springer, c2013. Description: xix, 1017 p.: ill. (some col.); 27 cm. ISBN: 9781461437932 (alk. paper) 1461437938 (alk. paper) LC classification: RC815.2 .P75 2013 Related names: Shaker, Reza. Partial contents: General Aspects of Deglutition. Overview of Deglutition and Digestion; Gustation, Olfaction and Deglutition; Coordination of Deglutition and Respiration; Airway Protective Mechanisms, Reciprocal Physiology of the Deglutitive Axis -- Central Control of Deglutition. Cerebral Cortical Control of Deglutition; Brainstem Control of Deglutition: Swallowing Pattern Generator; Brainstem Control of Deglutition: Brainstem Neural Circuits and Mediators Regulating Swallowing -- Preparatory/Oral Phase of Deglutition. Oral Phase Preparation and Propulsion: Anatomy, Physiology, Rheology, Mastication and Transport; Deglutitive Oral Pressure Phenomena; Effect of Aging on the Oral Phase of Deglutition; Nascent Oral Phase -- Pharyngeal Phase of Deglutition. Development, Anatomy and Physiology of the Pharynx; Development, Anatomy and Physiology of the Larynx; Development, Anatomy and Physiology of the Lungs; Effect of Aging of the Pharynx and the UES; Nascent Pharynx, Physiology, Reflexes -- UES and its Deglutitive Function. Development, Anatomy and Physiology of the Upper Esophageal Sphincter and Pharyngo-Esophageal Junction; Deglutitive Pharyngeal and UES Pressure Phenomena -- Esophageal Phase of Deglutition. Development, Anatomy and Physiology of the Esophagus; Normal Aging and the Esophagus; Nascent Esophagus, Sensory-Motor Physiology during Maturation -- Esophageal Motility and Its Deglutitive Function. Esophageal Motor Physiology;

Sphincter Mechanisms at the Esophago-Gastric Junction; Motility and Pressure Phenomena of the Esophagus -- Oral/Pharyngeal Phase Dysphagia. Symptom Indices for Dysphagia Assessment and Management; Cerebro-Vascular Accidents and Dysphagia; Progressive Neurologic Disease and Dysphagia (including Parkinson's Disease, Multiple Sclerosis, Amyotrophic Lateral Sclerosis, Myasthenia Gravis, Post Polio Syndrome); Disorders of Appetite, Eating and Swallowing in the Dementias; Dystrophies and Myopathies (including Muscular, Oculopharyngeal); Dysphagia Secondary to the Effects of Chemo and Radiation Therapy; Swallowing Syncope; Globus Pharyngeus; Deglutition in Patients with Tracheostomy, Nasogastric Tubes and Orogastric Tubes; Dysphagia Secondary to Systemic Diseases -- Upper Esophageal Sphincter Opening Dysfunction. Zenker's Diverticulum; Cricopharyngeal Bar; Cricopharyngeal Achalasia; UES Opening Muscle Dysfunction -- Esophageal Phase Dysphagia: Motor Disorders. Achalasia and Ineffective Esophageal Motility; Esophageal Spasm/Non-Cardiac Chest Pain Hypertensive Esophageal Peristalsis (Nutcracker Esophagus) Hypertensive Lower Esophageal Sphincter -- Esophageal Phase Dysphagia: Structural Abnormalities. Benign and Malignant Tumors of the Esophagus; Strictures, Rings, Webs (peptic, caustic, radiation, anastomotic); Esophageal Foreign Bodies: Food Impaction and Foreign Bodies; Post-Surgical Dysphagia: Post-Nissen Fundoplication, C-spine surgery, Thyroid surgery, Gastric Banding, Gastric Bypass; Drug-induced Esophageal Injury; Infectious Esophagitis; Eosinophilic Esophagitis; Gastroesophageal Reflux Disease; Barrett's Esophagus; Extraesophageal Manifestations of Reflux Disease and Dysphagia; Hiatal Hernia -- Eating Disorders. Psychogenic Dysphagia; Rumination Syndrome -- Treatment Options for Deglutition Disorders. Compensatory Management and Treatment in Dysphagia; Rehabilitative Treatments; Electrical Stimulation Treatment; Pharmacotherapy of UES Spastic Disorder; Open and Endoscopic Cricopharyngeal Myotomy; Surgical Treatment of Zenker's Diverticulum; Dilatations (UES, Esophagus, LES) Balloon Dilations,

Bougies; Esophageal Stenting for Relief of Dysphagia; Botulinum Toxin for LES Spastic Disorders; Surgical Treatment of Achalasia and Spastic Esophageal Disorders; Vocal Fold Medialization, Arytenoid Adduction, and Partial Pharyngectomy; Laryngohyoid Suspension; Surgical Management of Life-Threatening Aspiration; Anti-Reflux Surgery; Tube Feeding: Indications, Considerations and Technique. Subjects: Deglutition disorders. Deglutition. Deglutition Disorders--therapy. Deglutition--physiology. Deglutition Disorders--physiopathology. Notes: Includes bibliographical references and index. Dewey class no.: 616.3/23

Quagga and zebra mussels: biology, impacts, and control LCCN: : 2013017601 Zebra mussels. Quagga and zebra mussels: biology, impacts, and control / edited by Thomas F. Nalepa, Don W. Schloesser Edition: Second edition. Published/Produced: Boca Raton: CRC Press, Taylor & Francis Group, [2014] ©2014 Description: xxiv, 775 pages: illustrations (some color), maps (some color); 29 cm + 1 DVD-ROM (4 3/4 in.) ISBN: 9781439854365 (hardcover: acid-free paper) 143985436X (hardcover: acid-free paper) LC classification: QL430.7.D8 Z45 2014 Related names: Nalepa, T. F. Schloesser, Donald W. Scope and content: "The introduction and rapid spread of the zebra mussel in North American waters has caused great concern among industrial and recreational users of these waters. This bivalve mollusk is a biofouler that attaches to any firm substrate (e.g., rocks, piers, water intake pipes, boat hulls) and has already created significant problems for raw water users such as water treatment plants and power plants. Quagga and Zebra Mussels: Biology, Impacts and Control provides essential information regarding the biology of the zebra mussel in North America and Europe, presents case studies of environmental and industrial impacts, and outlines control strategies. Summary articles detail its life history, origins, and morphology. The book also examines techniques used to culture and maintain this organism in the laboratory. Thirty-two color plates illustrate some of the dramatic problems created by the explosive population growth of this species. Quagga and Zebra Mussels: Biology, Impacts, and Control is an important resource for ecologists, conservationists, environmental consultants, water quality engineers, regulatory officials, power utilities, and libraries"-- Provided by publisher. "The discovery of the zebra mussel, Dreissena polymorpha, in Lake St. Clair in 1988 signaled what was to become a major threat to the St. Lawrence Great Lakes. It became a matter of great concern when it combined with frazzle ice to clog the water intake pipes to Monroe, Michigan in 1989 and also when its rapid spread and exponential population growth threatened cooling water supplies to electric power plants, especially nuclear power plants, and industries around the Great Lakes. The zebra mussel also brought attention to aquatic organisms as invasive species. D. polymorpha and its related species, the quagga mussel D. rostriformis bugensis, would adversely impact other aquatic organisms and bring about changes in all the Great Lakes, except Lake Superior, by altering the food web, water clarity, water chemistry, and even the sediments and beaches. Furthermore, it appears that these changes may have altered the environment to favor the establishment of other invasive species"-- Provided by publisher. Contents: Preface / Thomas F. Nalepa and Don W. Schloesser -- Forward / Alfred M. Beeton -- My story on finding the first zebra mussel (Dreissena polymorpha) in North America / Sonya Gutschi Santavy -- In recognition: John Glenn sparks a giant leap for environmental protection / Allegra Cangelosi -- Chronological history of zebra and quagga mussels (Dreissenidae) in North America, 1988-2010 / Amy J. Benson -- Influence of environmental factors on zebra mussel population expansion in Lake Champlain, 1994-2010 / J. Ellen Marsden, Pete Stangel, and Angela D. Shambaugh -- Replacement of zebra mussels by quagga mussels in the Erie Canal, New York, USA / Kenton M. Stewart -- Invasion of quagga mussels (Dreissena rostriformis bugensis) to the mid-lake reef complex in Lake Michigan: a photographic montage / Jeffrey S. Houghton, Robert Paddock, and John Janssen -- Long-term change in the Hudson River's bivalve populations: a history of multiple invasions (and recovery?) / David L. Strayer and Heather M. Malcom -- Spread of the quagga mussel (Dreissena rostriformis bugensis) in Western Europe / Abraham bij de Vaate, Gerard van der Velde, Rob S.E.W. Leuven, and Katharina C.M. Heiler -- Origin and spread of quagga mussels (Dreissena rostriformis bugensis) in Eastern Europe with notes on size structure of populations / Marina I. Orlova -- Summary of zebra mussel (Dreissena polymorpha) in Polish lakes over the past 50 years with emphasis on the Masurian Lakes (northeastern Poland) / Krzysztof Lewandowski and Anna Staânczykowska -- One reporter's perspective on the invasion of dreissenid mussels in North America: reflections on the news media / Steve Pollick -- Early responses to zebra mussels in the Great Lakes: a journey from information vacuum to policy and regulation / Ronald W. Griffiths, Don W. Schloesser, and William P. Kovalak -- Catalyst for change: "The little dreissenid that did" (change national policy on aquatic invasive species) / David F. Reid and Dean Wilkinson -- Invading dreissenid mussels transform the 100-year-old International Joint Commission / Mark J. Burrows -- Eradication of zebra mussels (Dreissena polymorpha) from Millbrook Quarry, Virginia: rapid response in the real world / Raymond T. Fernald and Brian T. Watson -- Management and control of dreissenid mussels in water infrastructure facilities of the southwestern United States / Rajat K. Chakraborti, Sharook Madon, Jagjit Kaur, and Dale Gabel -- Impact of dreissenid mussels on the infrastructure of dams and hydroelectric power plants / Thomas H. Prescott, Renata Claudi, and Katherine L. Prescott -- Managing expansion of dreissenids within traditional parameters: the story of quagga mussels in Lake Mead National Recreation Area / Valerie Hickey -- Dreissenid mussels as sentinel biomonitors for human and zoonotic pathogens / David Bruce Conn, Frances E. Lucy, and Thaddeus K. Graczyk -- Contaminant concentrations in dreissenid mussels from the Laurentian Great Lakes: a summary of trends from the Mussel Watch Program / Kimani L. Kimbrough, W. Edward Johnson, Annie P. Jacob, and Gunnar G. Lauenstein -- Morphological variability of Dreissena polymorpha and Dreissena rostriformis bugensis (Mollusca: Bivalvia) / Vera

Pavlova and Yuri Izyumov -- Variation of the quagga mussel (Dreissena rostriformis bugensis) with emphasis on the deepwater morphotype in Lake Michigan / Thomas F. Nalepa, Vera Pavlova, Wai H. Wong, John Janssen, Jeffrey S. Houghton, and Kerrin Mabrey -- Behavior of juvenile and adult zebra mussels (Dreissena polymorpha) / Jaros±aw Kobak -- Antipredator strategy of zebra mussels (Dreissena polymorpha): from behavior to life history / Marcin Czarnoleski and Tomasz Mèuller -- Variation in predator-prey interactions between round gobies and dreissenid mussels / Christopher J. Houghton and John Janssen -- Density, growth, and reproduction of zebra mussels (Dreissena polymorpha) in two Oklahoma reservoirs / Chad J. Boeckman and Joseph R. Bidwell -- Limiting environmental factors and competitive interactions between zebra and quagga mussels in North America / David W. Garton, Robert McMahon, and Ann M. Stoeckmann -- Evolutionary, biogeographic, and population genetic relationships of dreissenid mussels, with revision of component taxa / Carol A. Stepien, Igor A. Grigorovich, Meredith A. Gray, Timothy J. Sullivan, Shane Yerga-Woolwine, and Gokhan Kalayci -- Effects of algal composition, seston stoichiometry, and feeding rate on zebra mussel (Dreissena polymorpha) nutrient excretion in two Laurentian Great Lakes / Thomas H. Johengen, Henry A. Vanderploeg, and James R. Liebig -- Chemical regulation of dreissenid reproduction / Donna R. Kashian and Jeffrey L. Ram -- Role of fluid dynamics in dreissenid mussel biology / Josef Daniel Ackerman -- Meta-analysis of dreissenid effects on freshwater ecosystems / Scott N. Higgins -- Effects of invasive quagga mussels (Dreissena rostriformis bugensis) on chlorophyll and water clarity in Lakes Mead and Havasu of the lower Colorado River Basin, 2007-2009 / Wai H. Wong, G. Chris Holdren, Todd Tietjen, Shawn Gerstenberger, Bryan Moore, Kent Turner, and Doyle C. Wilson -- Role of selective grazing by dreissenid mussels in promoting toxic Microcystis blooms and other changes in phytoplankton composition in the Great Lakes / Henry A. Vanderploeg, Alan E. Wilson, Thomas H. Johengen, Julianne Dyble Bressie, Orlando Sarnelle, James R. Liebig, Sander D.

Robinson, and Geoffrey P. Horst -- Trends in phytoplankton, zooplankton, and macroinvertebrates in Saginaw Bay relative to zebra mussel (Dreissena polymorpha) colonization: a generalized linear model approach / Sara Adlerstein, Thomas F. Nalepa, Henry A. Vanderploeg, and Gary L. Fahnenstiel -- Lake Michigan after dreissenid mussel invasion: water quality and food web changes during the late winter/spring isothermal period / Steven A. Pothoven and Gary L. Fahnenstiel -- Nutrient cycling by dreissenid mussels: controlling factors and ecosystem response / Harvey A. Bootsma and Qian Liao -- Benthification of freshwater lakes: exotic mussels turning ecosystems upside down / Christine M. Mayer, Lyubov E. Burlakova, Peter Eklèov, Dean Fitzgerald, Alexander Y. Karatayev, Stuart A. Ludsin, Scott Millard, Edward L. Mills, A.P. Ostapenya, Lars G. Rudstam, Bin Zhu, and Tataina V. Zhukova -- Variability of zebra mussel (Dreissena polymorpha) Impacts in the Shannon River system, Ireland / Dan Minchin and Anastasija Zaiko -- Impacts of Dreissena on benthic macroinvertebrate communities: predictable patterns revealed by invasion history / Jessica M. Ward and Anthony Ricciardi -- Interactions between an exotic ecosystem engineers (Dreissena spp.) and native burrowing mayflies (Hexagenia spp.) in soft sediments of western Lake Erie / Kristen M. DeVanna, Don W. Schloesser, Jonathan M. Bossenbroek, and Christine M. Mayer -- Zebra mussel impacts on unionids: a synthesis of trends in North America and Europe / Frances E. Lucy, Lyubov E. Burlakova, Alexander Y. Karatayev, Sergey E. Mastitsky, and David T. Zanatta -- Impacts of dreissenid mussels on the distribution and abundance of diving ducks on Lake St. Clair / David R. Luukkonen, Ernest N. Kafcas, Brendan T. Shirkey, and Scott R. Winterstein -- Context-dependent changes in lake whitefish populations associated with dreissenid invasion / Michael D. Rennie -- Effects of dreissenids on monitoring and management of fisheries in western Lake Erie / Martin A. Stapanian and Patrick M. Kocovsky -- General overview of zebra and quagga mussels: what we do and do not know / Alexander Y. Karatayev, Lyubov E. Burlakova, and Dianna K. Padilla --

Comparative role of dreissenids and other benthic invertebrates as links for type-E botulism transmission in the Great Lakes / Alicia Pâerez-Fuentetaja, Mark D. Clapsadl, and W. Theodore Lee -- A comparison of consumptive demand of Diporeia spp. and Dreissena in Lake Michigan based on bioenergetics models / Daniel J. Ryan, Thomas F. Nalepa, Lori N. Ivan, Maria S. Sepâulveda, and Tomas O. Hèoèok -- Variation in length-frequency distributions of zebra mussels (Dreissena polymorpha) within and between three Baltic Sea subregions: Szczecin Lagoon, Curonian Lagoon, and Gulf of Finland / Christiane Fenske, Anastasija Zaiko, Adam Woâzniczka, Sven Dahlke, and Marina I. Orlova -- A note on dreissenid mussels and historic shipwrecks / Russ Green -- Appendix: Narratives for video clips. Video clip 1. A visual documentation of the eradication of zebra mussels (Dreissena polymorpha) from Millbrook Quarry, Virginia / Raymond T. Fernald and Brian T. Watson; Video clip 2. Invasion of quagga mussels (Dreissena rostriformis bugensis) to the midlake reef complex in Lake Michigan: a video montage / Jeffrey S. Houghton, Robert Paddock, and John Janssen; Video clip 3. Close-up view of inhalant siphons of quagga mussels (Dreissena rostriformis bugensis, deepwater morph) on the midlake reef complex in Lake Michigan / Thomas F. Nalepa, Jeffrey S. Houghton, Robert Paddock, and John Janssen; Video clip 4. Visual documentation of quagga mussels (Dreissena rostriformis bugensis) at two depths in southeastern Lake Michigan / Russ Miller, Nathan Hawley, and Steven A. Ruberg; Video clip 5. Zebra mussel movements on the bottom of Lake Michigan / Barry M. Lesht and Nathan Hawley; Video clip 6. Behavior of zebra mussels exposed to Microcystis colonies from natural seston and laboratory cultures / Henry A. Vanderploeg and J. Rudi Strickler; Video clip 7. Visual evidence a native mussel population (Unionidae: Bivalvia) in the St. Clair River (Laurentian Great Lakes) has survived despite the presence of Dreissena / Greg Lashbrook and Kathy Johnson -- Postlude-synopsis / Thomas F. Nalepa and Don W. Schloesser.
Subjects: Zebra mussel. Quagga mussel. Zebra mussel--Control. Quagga mussel--Control. Zebra mussel--Environmental aspects. Quagga mussel--Environmental

aspects. NATURE / Ecology. SCIENCE / Life Sciences / Biology / Marine Biology. TECHNOLOGY & ENGINEERING / Environmental / Water Supply. Notes: "A CRC title, part of the Taylor & Francis imprint, a member of the Taylor & Francis Group, the academic division of T&F Informa plc." First edition published with title: Zebra mussels. c1993. Includes bibliographical references and index. Dewey class no.: 594/.4

Techniques of botulinum toxin injections in the head and neck LCCN: 2012011987 Benninger, Michael S. Techniques of botulinum toxin injections in the head and neck / Michael S. Benninger and P. Daniel Knott. Published/Created: San Diego, CA: Plural Pub., c2012. Projected pub date: 1111 Description: p.; cm. ISBN: 9781597564427 (alk. paper) 1597564427 (alk. paper) Related names: Knott, P. Daniel (Philip Daniel) Contents: Botox in medical applications: history, types of toxin, and doses / Anne Hseu -- Laryngeal dystonias / Michael S. Benninger -- Blepharospasm / Michael S. Benninger -- Hemifacial spasm / Michael S. Benninger -- Spasmodic torticollis or cervical dystonia / Michael S. Benninger -- Oromandibular dystonia / Michael S. Benninger -- Headaches / Michael S. Benninger -- Cricopharyngeus muscle dysfunction / Michael S. Benninger -- Salivary gland injections / Michael S. Benninger -- Frey's syndrome / Peter C. Revenaugh -- Theory and principles in aesthetic use / P. Daniel Knott -- Glabella / P. Daniel Knott -- Forehead treatment and brow repositioning / P. Daniel Knott -- Periorbital rejuvenation / Andrea Jarchow -- Perioral and cervical refinement / P. Daniel Knott -- Treatment of facial paralysis and synkinesis / P. Daniel Knott. Subjects: Botulinum Toxins--therapeutic use. Dystonia--drug therapy. Head. Neck. Synkinesis--drug therapy. Notes: Includes bibliographical references and index. Dewey class no.: 615.9/5

The case of the rusty nail LCCN: 2011029275 Faulk, Michelle. The case of the rusty nail / Michelle Faulk. Published/Created: Berkeley Heights, NJ: Enslow Publishers, c2013. Description: 48 p.: col. ill.; 24 cm. ISBN: 9780766039490 LC classification: RC359.5 .F38 2013 Summary: "Learn about diseases and their symptoms such as tetnus, West Nile virus, and Botulism among others"--Provided by publisher. Subjects: Nervous system--Infections--Juvenile literature. Notes: Includes bibliographical references (p. 47) and index. Series: Body system disease investigations Dewey class no.: 616.9/3

Index

Index

D

E

F

G

H

T

U

V

W

Z